Study Guide

to accompany

Wong's Essentials of Pediatric Nursing

7th Edition

Study Guide

to accompany

Wong's Essentials of Pediatric Nursing

7th Edition

Angela C. Murphy, PhD, RN
Professor of Pediatric Nursing (retired)
Rhode Island College
Providence, Rhode Island

ELSEVIER
MOSBY

ELSEVIER
MOSBY

11830 Westline Industrial Dr.
St. Louis, Missouri 63146

STUDY GUIDE TO ACCOMPANY   ISBN 0-323-03230-3
WONG'S ESSENTIALS OF PEDIATRIC NURSING
SEVENTH EDITION
Copyright © 2005, 2001, 1997, 1993, 1989   Mosby, Inc.   All rights reserved.

Although for mechanical reasons all pages of this publication are perforated, only those pages imprinted
with a Mosby, Inc. copyright notice are intended for removal.

Notice

Pediatric nursing is an ever-changing field. Standard safety precautions must be followed, but as new
research and clinical experience broaden our knowledge, changes in treatment and drug therapy may
become necessary or appropriate. Readers are advised to check the most current product information provided by the manufacturer of each drug to be administered to verify the recommended dose, the method and
duration of administration, and contraindications. It is the responsibility of the licensed prescriber, relying
on experience and knowledge of the patient, to determine dosages and the best treatment for each individual
patient. Neither the publisher nor the editor assumes any liability for any injury and/or damage to persons
or property arising from this publication.

International Standard Book Number 0-323-03230-3

Executive Editor: *Loren Wilson*
Senior Developmental Editor: *Michele D. Hayden*
Project Manager: *Ann Rogers*

Printed in the United States of America

Last digit is the print number: 9   8   7   6   5   4   3   2   1

Acknowledgements

I extend my appreciation and thanks to my daughter, Maia, for her competent and efficient assistance in the editing and preparation of the manuscript for this Study Guide. A special note of thanks to my husband, whose support, encouragement, and daily contributions made the final completion of this manuscript possible.

Contents

Unit Eight—Impact of Hospitalization on the Child and Family

Unit Nine—The Child with Problems Related to the Transfer of Oxygen and Nutrients

Unit Ten—The Child with Problems Related to the Production and Circulation of Blood

Unit Eleven—The Child With a Disturbance of Regulatory Mechanisms

Unit Twelve—Th e Child with a Problem that Interferes with Physical Mobility

Perspectives of Pediatric Nursing

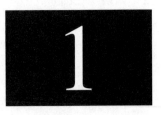

The content of Chapter 1 provides an overview of the nursing care of children from a child-centered perspective that views children as unique individuals rather than miniature adults. The multifaceted roles of the pediatric nurse are explored. The focus of care, whether treating or preventing illness, is child-centered and family-centered. At the completion of this chapter, the student will be able to use the nursing process and critical thinking skills to deliver individualized and effective nursing care to children and their families.

REVIEW OF ESSENTIAL CONCEPTS

Health

1. The World Health Organization (WHO) defines *health* as:

2. "Healthy People 2010" has two goals for Public Health in America; these are:

   a.

   b.

Mortality

3. Define *infant mortality*.

4. The United States lags behind other countries of the world in infant mortality rate. In 1999, the United States

   ranked _____ among the 25 nations with the lowest infant death rates.

5. The country with the lowest infant mortality rate is _____ _____.

6. _____ _____ _____ is considered the major determinant of neonatal death in technologically developed countries.

7. The major cause of death for children over the age of 1 year is _____ _____.

Morbidity

8. The term *morbidity* is defined as:
   a. the number of individuals who have died over a specific period of time.
   b. the prevalence of a specific illness in the population at a particular time.
   c. disease occurring with greater frequency than the number of expected cases in a community.
   d. disease occurring regularly within a geographic location.

9. The most common acute childhood illness is:
   a. cancer.
   b. respiratory illness.
   c. tonsillitis.
   d. enuresis.

10. Behavioral, social, and educational problems are sometimes referred to as the _____ _____.

Child Health Care in the United States

11. _____ _____, who is known as the Father of Pediatrics, influenced the beginning of the discipline of pediatrics in the 1800s.

12. _____ _____ is the founder of public health or community nursing services and established the role of the first school nurse.

13. The research findings of _____ and _____ highlighted the effects of isolation and maternal deprivation on institutionalized children and thus stimulated change in how hospitalized children are treated.

14. Match each federal program for maternal and child health with its description.

   a. ___ Medicaid

   b. ___ Aid to Families with Dependent Children (AFDC)

   c. ___ Social Services Block Grant

   d. ___ Women, Infants, and Children (WIC)

   e. ___ Education for All Handicapped Children Act (P.L. 94-142 and P.L. 99-457)

   f. ___ Family and Medical Leave Act (FMLA)

   1. Free appropriate public education to handicapped children from ages 3 to 21 years. Federal funding to support early intervention services for handicapped infants and toddlers and their families.

   2. Under Title XIX, reduces financial barrier to health care for the poor.

   3. Under Title XX, provides states with funds for child daycare, protective and emergency services, as well as counseling, family planning, home-based services, adoption and foster care services.

   4. Enable states to aid needy children without fathers.

   5. Allows employees up to 12 weeks of unpaid leave from their job to care for a newborn or child, parent or spouse who is seriously ill.

   6. Provides nutritious food and nutrition education to low-income, pregnant, postpartum, and lactating women and infants and children up to age 5 years. Includes Food Stamps and School Lunch Programs.

15. The two basic concepts of family-centered care are:
   a. enabling and empowerment.
   b. encouragement and facilitation.
   c. policy and practice.
   d. partnership and caring.

16. Case management was developed as an approach to _____ care and _____ costs, using timelines in _____ plans.

17. The AHCPR has developed _____ _____ _____ relevant to pediatric practice.

18. Identify the major roles of the pediatric nurse.

    a.

    b.

    c.

    d.

    e.

    f.

    g.

    h.

    i.

    j.

19. The shift in focus from treatment of disease to promotion of health will expand the nurse's role in ambula-

    tory care. The portions of the role that will receive the major emphasis are _____ and

    _____ _____.

Critical Thinking and the Process of Nursing Children and Families

20. Define *critical thinking*.

21. Define the nursing process.

22. List the five steps of the nursing process.

    a.

    b.

    c.

d.

e.

23. Assessment is a continuous process that operates at all phases of problem solving and is the

_____ of _____ _____.

24. The second stage in the nursing process requires that the nurse interpret the data that was assessed and identify problems. These problems, or clinical judgments, are termed _____ _____.

25. The three components of nursing diagnosis are: _____ _____; _____;

_____ and _____.

26. Match each of the following definitions with the appropriate term.

a. ____ Problem statement

b. ____ Etiology

c. ____ Signs and symptoms

1. Describes the child's response to health pattern deficits in the child, family, or community.

2. The cluster of cues and/or defining characteristics that are derived from the patient assessment.

3. Describes the physiologic, situational, and maturational factors that cause the problem or influence its development.

27. Nursing practice consists of three dimensions. They are _____, _____, and

_____ activities.

28. What is (are) established in the planning stage of the nursing process?

29. Define the two types of nursing care plans.

a. Standard care plans

b. Individualized care plans

30. The third step in the nursing process is _____, when the nurse and patient act to achieve the specific outcome or goal.

31. The last step in the nursing process is _____. This is when the nurse determines whether the

_____ has been met or whether the plan must be modified.

APPLYING CRITICAL THINKING TO NURSING PRACTICE

A. Spend a day following a nurse in a pediatric unit of an acute care facility.

1. Briefly describe and give examples of the roles of the pediatric nurse in a pediatric unit.

a. Family advocacy

b. Disease prevention/health promotion

c. Restorative role

d. Coordination/collaboration

e. Ethical decision making

f. Research

B. You observe the care of a group of four children on an acute care unit of a children's hospital for one shift. Which principle of family-centered care is being applied or violated in the following examples?

1. The father of a child can visit for only two hours. During this time, the nurse decides to give the child's unscheduled 30-minute treatment and asks the father to step outside the room.

2. The posted visiting hours are noon to 8 p.m. for families, and no children under 14 years of age are allowed.

3. A mother is doing a dressing on her child's leg. The nurse is observing and assisting as necessary.

4. The nurse would like to perform the morning bath on a child. The mother is just awakening. The nurse asks the mother whether she would prefer this activity to occur now or at a more convenient time for her and the child.

C. Spend a morning in a pediatric unit and complete a comprehensive assessment of one child and his or her family.

1. Identify whether the following characteristic of "assessment" describes a standardized or individualized care plan: Information is specific to both identified problem and the child and family.

2. Identify whether the following characteristic of "nursing diagnosis" describes a standardized or individualized care plan: All probable nursing diagnoses with general etiologic factors are considered.

3. Identify whether the following characteristic of "planning" describes a standardized or individualized care plan: Goals are specific and reflect patient outcomes.

4. Identify whether the following characteristic of "implementation" describes a standardized or individualized care plan: Nursing interventions are specific and provide direction for nursing care of individual patient.

5. Identify whether the following characteristic of "evaluation" describes a standardized or individualized care plan: Progress the patient is expected to make is identified.

Community-Based Nursing Care of the Child and Family

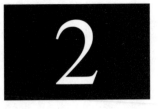

Chapter 2 explores the role of the nurse in the multidisciplinary approach to care of children and families in the community setting. The concepts and principles of community health nursing are explored. The components of the community nursing process are explained and contrasted with the nursing process used for an individual child or family. Planning and evaluation of health programs are explained. Collaboration of the nurse with members of the community is stressed as essential to the success of any health program designed to increase the health status of the community.

REVIEW OF ESSENTIAL CONCEPTS

Community Concepts

1. According to Anderson and McFarlane (2000), *community* is defined as:

2. Does the definition "groups of people toward whom health care workers direct their activities to improve the health status of individuals in the group" describe *populations* or *target populations*?

3. According to Allender and Spradley (2001) and Williams (2000), *community health nursing* is defined as:

4. Demography is the study of _____ characteristics and includes age, gender, _____/

   _____, _____ _____, and education.

5. *Risk* is defined as:

6. Define *epidemiology*.

7. Morbidity (disease and injury) is reported using two types of rates. What are they?

8. _____ measures the occurrence of new events in a population during a period of time.

   _____ measures existing events in a population during a period of time.

9. The Epidemiologic Triangle is formed by three factors whose interrelationship alters the risk for acquiring a disease or condition; they are _____, _____, and _____.

10. Match each level of prevention with its descriptions.

    a. ____ Primary prevention

    b. ____ Secondary prevention

    c. ____ Tertiary prevention

    1. Interventions that promote health and protect children from disease or injury. Examples are: well-child care clinics, immunization programs, safety programs, sanitation programs, and parenting classes.

    2. Interventions that optimize function for children with disability or chronic disease. Examples are: rehabilitation and management programs for asthma, sickle cell disease, anorexia, and special education programs for children.

    3. Interventions that promote early detection and treatment of illness or efforts to prevent the spread of contagious diseases, progression of disease, or disability. Examples are: tuberculosis and lead screening, early intervention developmental services, mental health counseling for stressful events.

11. Screening for disease must be carefully planned to ensure the _____ of screening exceed the risks and cost.

12. Economic evaluation provides _____ _____ to establish the value of a program to the community.

Community Nursing Process

13. In community nursing the focus of the nursing process shifts from the individual child and family to the

    _____ or target population.

14. A community needs assessment requires the collection of both _____ and _____ information about a community.

15. Just as a physical assessment is organized around the body systems, the community needs assessment can be

    organized around _____ _____.

16. Based on an analysis of the community assessment, the nurse formulates a _____

    _____ _____.

17. In the planning phase of the community nursing process, the nurse collaborates with community members to

    develop a _____ to address the needs and problems of the target population.

18. Community interventions often are offered in the form of _____ _____.

19. Evaluation identifies whether the _____ and _____ _____ of the health
    program were met.

APPLYING CRITICAL THINKING TO NURSING PRACTICE

A. Spend a day following a nurse in an elementary school. Identify which "level of prevention" the following
   activities of the nurse are illustrating.

   1. Evaluating the immunization status of the children entering the first grade and encouraging compliance
      with requirements.

   2. Teaching the third-grade students about the importance of bicycle helmets.

   3. Assisting a fourth-grade child in complying with the medication schedule for the child's asthma.

   4. Consulting with the classroom teacher regarding health education of a special education child in the third
      grade.

   5. Organizing and conducting a support group for children of divorced parents.

   6. Preventing the return to school of a child with open sores from chicken pox.

B. You are accompanying a community health nurse who, together with a community group, is conducting a
   community needs assessment.

   1. What are the eight community systems that the nurse needs to examine?

   2. Give an example of how the nurse would gather subjective information about the community.

3. What are the sources of objective data about the community that the nurse could access?

4. After analyzing the assessment data, the nurse and the community group identify that the compliance with immunization schedules of children under 2 years old is only 50 percent. Based on this data, what is the community nursing diagnosis?

5. State an example of a short-term goal to address this nursing diagnosis.

6. The group plans to achieve this goal. Program objectives are set. In order to evaluate the goals and objectives of the program, the nurse would use the Donabedian model. Explain the approach of this model.

Family Influences on Child Health Promotion

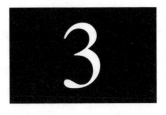

Chapter 3 provides an overview of family and parenting influences on health promotion of children. Theories of family and different family structures are explored. The role transition of new parents and the effect of family size on personality development are discussed. Since families assume the primary responsibility for child rearing and socialization, students need to recognize the impact of the family on the developing child. At the completion of this chapter, the student will have knowledge of a variety of family situations that will serve as a foundation for the development of appropriate nursing strategies.

REVIEW OF ESSENTIAL CONCEPTS

General Concepts

1. There is no universal definition of family; a family is:

2. Explain the following three major family theories:

   a. Family System Theory

   b. Family Stress Theory

   c. Developmental Theory

Family Structure and Function

3. Match the following family structures with the appropriate definition.

   a. ____ Traditional nuclear

   b. ____ Single parent

   c. ____ Blended

   d. ____ Extended

   e. ____ Gay/lesbian

1. One parent, one or more children, and one or more members (related or unrelated) other than a parent or sibling.

2. A man or woman alone as head of a household as a result of divorce, death, desertion, illegitimacy, or adoption.

3. A common-law tie between two persons of the same sex who have children.

4. A man, his wife, and their children who live in a common household.

5. Married adults, one or both of whose children from a previous marriage reside in the household.

Family Roles and Relationships

4. Roles are learned through the _____ process.

5. Identify the four elements of family configuration that influence child development.

   a.

   b.

   c.

   d.

6. To differentiate between small and large families, identify whether the following statements are true or false.

   a.   T   F   Emphasis is placed on the individual development of the child in the small family.

   b.   T   F   Children in large families are unable to adjust to a variety of changes and crises.

   c.   T   F   Adolescents from a large family are often more peer-oriented than family-oriented.

7. Ordinal position in a family may influence a child's personality development. Are the following statements true or false?

   a.   T   F   Only children resemble middle children.

   b.   T   F   First-born children are more achievement-oriented and more dominant.

   c.   T   F   Youngest children are more dependent than first-born children.

   d.   T   F   Middle children are able to compromise and be adaptable.

Parenting

8. Identify the three basic goals of parenting.

    a.

    b.

    c.

9. Briefly identify the five factors that can influence the parental role.

    a.

    b.

    c.

    d.

    e.

10. Differentiate among the following three styles of parental control.

    a. Authoritarian (dictatorial)

    b. Permissive (laissez-faire)

    c. Authoritative (democratic)

11. Identify the seven most common strategies (types) for discipline.

    a.

    b.

    c.

    d.

    e.

    f.

    g.

12. Match each guideline for implementing discipline with its explanation.

    a. ___ Consistency   1. Follow through with the details of discipline.

    b. ___ Timing   2. Always disapprove of the behavior, not the child.

    c. ___ Commitment   3. Implement disciplinary action exactly as agreed upon for each infraction.

    d. ___ Flexibility

    e. ___ Behavior orientation   4. Once the discipline is administered, consider the child as having a "clean slate."

    f. ___ Termination   5. Choose disciplinary strategies that are appropriate to the child's age and temperament and the severity of the misbehavior.

                                       6. Initiate discipline as soon as the child misbehaves.

Special Parenting Situations

13. State the three areas of concern for adoptive parents.

    a.

    b.

    c.

14. Identify the factors that will influence the impact of divorce on children.

    a.

    b.

    c.

    d.

15. T   F   It has been determined that at least half the children born in the 1990s in the United States will spend some time in a single-parent home.

16. The Family and Medical Leave Act (FMLA) provides for:

APPLYING CRITICAL THINKING TO NURSING PRACTICE

A. Interview an expectant couple and parents with adolescent children to contrast their views of parenthood. Answer the following questions and include the parents' responses to illustrate these concepts.

    1. According to Duvall's Development Stages of the Family Theory, what are the tasks for each of the following families? Are these families successful in accomplishing these tasks?

        a. Expectant couple

        b. Parents of adolescent children

    2. What factors affect the transition to parenthood?

B. After talking with children from a variety of families, answer the following questions that deal with the effects of different family structures on child development. Include specific examples to illustrate these concepts.

    1. What events might alter family structure?

    2. What implication does an alteration in composition have for the family and child?

    3. List the qualities of strong families, regardless of their configuration.

        a.

        b.

        c.

        d.

        e.

f.

g.

h.

i.

j.

k.

l.

C.   Talk to a single parent, as a result of divorce, to assess problem areas. Answer the following questions.

1. What changes or feelings accompany single parenthood?

2. The impact of divorce on the child depends on a variety of factors. What are they?

a.

b.

c.

d.

D.   Interview a couple who are dual-career parents to assess problem areas. Answer the following questions and include specific parental responses.

1. Identify some of the major problems associated with dual-career families.

Social, Cultural, and Religious Influences on Child Health Promotion

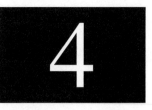

Chapter 4 provides an overview of the social, cultural, religious, and economic factors influencing the growth and development of children in the United States. The influence of cultural and religious beliefs on health care practices is discussed at length. At the completion of this chapter, the student will have a knowledge of the social, economic, cultural, and religious influences that affect the health promotion of the child. This knowledge will enable the student to adapt the delivery of nursing care to the unique needs of the child and family.

REVIEW OF ESSENTIAL CONCEPTS

Culture

1. Match each concept with its definition.

   a. ___ Culture

   b. ___ Race

   c. ___ Ethnicity

   d. ___ Socialization

   1. The process by which children acquire the competencies, values, and expectations of a given society.

   2. A pattern of assumptions, beliefs, and practices that unconsciously frames or guides the outlook and decisions of a group of people.

   3. The affiliation of a set of persons who share a unique cultural, social, and linguistic heritage.

   4. A division of human beings possessing traits that are transmissible by descent and sufficient to characterize it as a distinct human type.

2. A social group consists of a system of roles carried out in both primary and secondary groups.

   a. A primary group is characterized by:

   b. A secondary group is characterized by:

3. Define *ethnicity*.

17

4. The term _____ refers to the emotional attitude that one's own ethnic group is superior to others; that one's values, beliefs, and perceptions are the correct ones; and that the group's ways of living and behaving are the best way.

5. The term *visible poverty* refers to:

6. The term *invisible poverty* refers to:

7. Low-income working families are raising approximately _____% of America's children.

8. A large group of homeless children described as runaways or throwaways are _____.

9. _____ families are subject to inadequate sanitation, substandard housing, social isolation, and a lack of educational and medical facilities.

10. Next to the family, the _____ exert the major force in providing continuity between generations by conveying a vast amount of culture from the older members to the young.

11. There are four categories of external assets that youth receive from the community. List them.

   a.

   b.

   c.

   d.

12. Identify four functions of peer cultures.

   a.

   b.

   c.

   d.

13. Define the term *biculturation*.

14. Family life in North America is characterized by increasing _____ and _____ mobility.

15. Define the term *cultural shock*.

Cultural/Religious Influences on Health Care

16. Match each common disease or disorder with the ethnic or cultural group it affects.

    a. ___ Type 2 diabetes   1. Ashkenasi Jewish

    b. ___ Tay-Sachs disease   2. Blacks

    c. ___ Cystic fibrosis   3. Whites

    d. ___ Sickle cell disease   4. Native Americans

17. The most overwhelming adverse influence on the health of children is _____ status.

18. _____ _____ is the concept that any behavior must be judged first in relation to the context of the culture in which it occurs.

19. Identify the areas in which there might be a conflict of values and customs for the nurse interacting with a child and family from a different cultural or ethnic group.

    a.

    b.

    c.

    d.

    e.

    f.

    g.

    h.

    i.

    j.

    k.

    l.

    m.

    n.

20. Match the following religious beliefs with the religion they represent.

    a. ____ Oppose human intervention with drugs
        or other therapies.

    b. ____ Are taught not to refuse treatment in the
        belief that Allah will take care of them.

    c. ____ Opposed to blood transfusions.

    d. ____ May resist surgical procedures during
        Sabbath.

    e. ____ Traditional church teaching does not
        approve of contraceptives or abortion.

    1. Roman Catholicism

    2. Judaism

    3. Christian Science

    4. Islam (Muslim/Moslem)

    5. Jehovah's Witness

21. Which three religious groups have beliefs that significantly affect their health practices and their willingness
    to receive treatment?

    a.

    b.

    c.

22. Match the following cultural characteristics with the culture they represent.

    a. ____ Goal of therapy is to restore balance of
        Yin and Yang.

    b. ____ Illness classified as natural or unnatural.
        Self-care and folk medicine very prevalent.

    c. ____ Subscribe to hot-cold theory of causation
        of illness.

    d. ____ Believe health is state of harmony with
        nature and universe

    1. Native Americans

    2. African Americans

    3. Asian Americans

    4. Puerto Ricans

APPLYING CRITICAL THINKING TO NURSING PRACTICE

A. Interview parents from a variety of cultural, ethnic, economic, and religious backgrounds to determine the
   differences in child-rearing practices. Answer the following questions and include specific parental
   responses that illustrate the concepts.

   1. What are some of the subcultural influences that may affect this family's child-rearing practices?

      a.

      b.

      c.

      d.

e.

f.

g.

2. Briefly describe the influence that the following aspects of contemporary American culture have on child development.

   a. An optimistic view of the world and belief that things can be better

   b. Increasing geographic and economic mobility

   c. A basically nuclear-family orientation

B. Spend a day in a health care center that serves a multicultural community. Answer the following questions and include specific observations as appropriate.

   1. What factors increase a child's susceptibility to health problems?

      a. Hereditary factors

      b. Socioeconomic factors

   2. How do the following factors contribute to the development of health problems in children from lower socioeconomic classes?

      a. Inadequate funds for food

      b. Lack of funds and access to health care

    c. Poor sanitation and crowded living conditions

  3. Why should nurses working in a multicultural community be aware of their own attitudes and values?

  4. What three areas of religious belief should be evaluated when assessing health care practices?

    a.

    b.

    c.

C. Spend a morning in an inner-city health clinic. Observe the multicultural patient's interaction with health care personnel. In what areas might you notice conflict between the health care personnel and the patients?

  1. Orientation to time

  2. Parental expectations

  3. Approach to child

  4. Involvement of family

  5. Communication difficulties

  6. Health beliefs and practices

Developmental Influences on Child Health Promotion

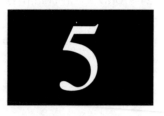

Chapter 5 provides an overview of the physiologic, psychologic, environmental, and social factors influencing the growth and development process. The role of play in the development of the child is explored. Upon completion of this chapter, the student should be aware of the theoretical foundations of all areas of development. This knowledge will serve as a basis for nursing interventions to meet the complex needs of the developing child.

REVIEW OF ESSENTIAL CONCEPTS

Growth and Development

1. Match each term with its definition.

   a. ____ Growth

   b. ____ Maturation

   c. ____ Development

   d. ____ Differentiation

   1. An increase in competence, adaptability, and aging.

   2. A gradual growth and expansion involving a change from lower to more advanced stages of complexity.

   3. An increase in number and size of cells as they divide and synthesize new proteins; results in increased size and weight of the whole or any of its parts.

   4. A biologic description of the processes by which early cells and structures are modified and altered to achieve specific, characteristic physical and chemical properties.

2. A _____ _____ is a set of skills and competencies peculiar to each developmental stage that children must master.

3. Fill in the ages denoted by each of the following periods of development.

   a. Prenatal period

   b. Neonatal period

   c. Infancy

   d. Toddler period

   e. Preschool period

   f. Middle childhood or school age

   g. Prepubertal

   h. Adolescence

23

4. List the three directional trends in growth and development.

   a.

   b.

   c.

5. Those times in the lifetime of an organism when it is more vulnerable to positive or negative influences are

   called _____ _____.

6. Growth and development proceeds in _____ patterns of direction, sequence, and pace.

7. T F The rate of growth is the same for all children.

8. For each of the following stages of development, match the body part in which growth predominates.

   a. ___ Prenatal   1. Trunk

   b. ___ Infancy   2. Head

   c. ___ Early and middle childhood   3. Shoulder and hip breadth

   d. ___ Adolescence   4. Legs

9. _____ the child's height at age 2 years to estimate how tall he/she will be as an adult.

10. Describe changes in birth weight typically seen by 4 to 7 months of age; by the end of the first year; and by the end of the second year.

11. No new nerve cells appear after the _____ month of fetal life.

12. T F Lymphoid tissue follows a growth pattern that is similar to that of other body tissues.

13. The basal caloric requirement for infants is about _____ kcal/kg of body weight and decreases to

    somewhere between _____ and _____ kcal/kg at maturity.

14. Identify the temperamental category that is described by each of the following.

    a. Highly active, irritable, and irregular in habits; adapts slowly to routines, people, situations

    b. Reacts negatively and with mild intensity to new stimuli; quite inactive and moody but shows only moderate irregularity in functions

    c. Even-tempered, regular, and predictable in habits; has positive approach to new stimuli; open and adaptable to change

Development of Personality and Mental Function

15. Match the five stages of psychosexual development (Freud) with the ages encompassed by each.

    a. ____ Oral stage   1. 1 to 3 years

    b. ____ Anal stage   2. Birth to 1 year

    c. ____ Phallic stage   3. 3 to 6 years

    d. ____ Latency period   4. 6 to 12 years

    e. ____ Genital stage   5. 12 to 18 years

16. For each of the following age groups, identify Erikson's stage of psychosocial development.

    a. Birth to 1 year

    b. 1 to 3 years

    c. 3 to 6 years

    d. 6 to 12 years

    e. 12 to 18 years

17. Match each stage of cognitive development (Piaget) with its defining characteristics (more than one answer may apply).

    a. ____ Sensorimotor stage (birth to 2 years)

    b. ____ Preoperational stage (2 to 7 years)

    c. ____ Concrete operations (7 to 11 years)

    d. ____ Formal operations (11 to 15 years)

    1. Predominant characteristic is egocentrism.

    2. Thought is characterized by adaptability and flexibility.

    3. Child progresses from reflex activity to imitative behavior.

    4. Thought becomes increasingly logical and coherent; conservation is developed; problems are solved in a concrete, systematic fashion.

    5. Child begins to develop a sense of self as he or she differentiates self from environment.

    6. Child can think in abstract terms, use abstract symbols, and draw logical conclusions.

    7. Child considers points of view other than his or her own; thinking becomes socialized.

    8. Child is unable to see things from any perspective other than his or her own; thinking is concrete.

18. At all stages of language development, a child's _____ vocabulary is greater than their

    _____ vocabulary.

19. Identify the stage of moral development (Kohlberg) that is described by each of the following statements.

   a. Children conform to rules imposed by authority figures and are culturally oriented to the labels of good/bad and right/wrong.

   b. Children endeavor to define moral values and principles that are agreed upon by the entire society. Emphasis is on the possibility for changing law in terms of societal needs.

   c. Children are concerned with conformity and loyalty and actively maintaining, supporting, and justifying the social order.

20. Define the term *self-concept*.

21. A vital component of self-concept is the subjective concepts and attitudes that individuals have toward their own bodies; this is termed _____ _____.

22. The term _____-_____ refers to a personal, subjective judgment of one's worthiness derived from the immediate environment and the individual's perception of how he or she is valued by others.

Role of Play in Development

23. Match each type of play with its defining characteristics.

   a. ____ Solitary play

   b. ____ Cooperative play

   c. ____ Onlooker play

   d. ____ Associative play

   e. ____ Parallel play

   1. Child watches what other children are doing but makes no attempt to enter into the play activity.

   2. Child plays alone and independently with toys different from those of other children within the same area.

   3. Child plays independently among other children with toys that are like those that the children around him or her are using, neither influencing nor being influenced by them.

   4. Child plays with other children, engaging in a similar or identical activity in which there is no organization, division of labor, or mutual goal.

   5. Child plays in a group with other children with discussion and planning of activities for accomplishing an end.

24. List the seven functions that play serves to develop throughout childhood.

    a.

    b.

    c.

    d.

    e.

    f.

    g.

Selected Factors That Influence Development

25. T   F   The single most important influence on growth is nutrition.

26. The most prominent feature of emotional deprivation, particularly during the first year, is _____

    _____.

27. The _____ _____ of children's families has a significant impact on growth and development.

28. Stress in childhood has been defined by Masten and others (1988) as:

29. _____ has become one of the most significant socializing agents in the lives of young children.

30. List five important ideas to teach children and adolescents about television.

    a.

    b.

    c.

    d.

    e.

31. Although computers have increased the interactive learning of children, there are dangers. Nurses should

    encourage parents to be _____ about their children's Internet activities in order to ensure their safety.

APPLYING CRITICAL THINKING TO NURSING PRACTICE

A. Sean, 2 years old, comes into the clinic for a well-child visit. The nurse will assess Sean's growth and development. Interpret the following assessment data.

1. Sean weighed 7 pounds 2 ounces at birth. His weight today is 21 pounds 2 ounces. Is this a normal increase? If not, what would be the expected gain?

2. Sean's mother wants to know whether his height at this age has any significance for his adult height. What would you tell her?

3. The nurse observes Sean interacting with his mother. After the assessment Sean insists on putting his clothes on himself. His mother patiently allows him to do this. Is this appropriate developmental behavior? Did Sean's mother respond appropriately?

B. Observe a child from each age group: infant, toddler, preschool, school-age, and adolescent.

1. Why is it necessary to have an understanding of patterns of development before assessing a child's developmental status?

2. Identify the psychosocial conflict of each age group and provide a specific intervention that will assist in the resolution of this conflict (Erikson).

   a. Infant

   b. Toddler

   c. Preschool

   d. School-age

   e. Adolescent

3. What behavior might be observed in each age group that would indicate the level of spiritual development?

   a. Infant

   b. Toddler

   c. Preschool

   d. School-age

   e. Adolescent

C. Interview the parents of a newborn regarding the infant's temperament.

   1. What is the significance of assessing a child's temperament?

   2. Identify behavioral characteristics that would indicate the temperament pattern of each of the following children.

      a. The easy child

      b. The difficult child

D. Attend a PTA meeting at your local elementary school.

   1. If you are asked to cite guidelines related to TV viewing for children this age, what guidelines would you present to this group?

      a.

      b.

      c.

      d.

      e.

      f.

      g.

h.

i.

j.

k.

l.

m.

n.

o.

p.

q.

r.

s.

t.

Communication and Health Assessment of the Child and Family

Chapter 6 introduces the essential components of communication in the nursing care of children and their families. Communication is an essential skill in the assessment process and is crucial to the establishment of a trusting relationship with children and their families. Guidelines for taking a health history and nutritional assessment are presented. At the completion of this chapter, the student should have knowledge of the elements of the communication process with children and their families and will be able to apply this knowledge in clinical practice.

REVIEW OF ESSENTIAL CONCEPTS

Communication

1. There are three forms of communication. Define each of these forms.

    a. Verbal communication

    b. Nonverbal communication

    c. Abstract communication

Guidelines for Communication and Interviewing

2. The place where the interview occurs is almost as important as the interview itself. What characteristics contribute to an effective setting?

3. _____ via telephone report occurs when the nurse assesses a child's symptoms and makes a clinical judgment on the urgency and type of treatment needed.

Communicating With Families

4. Various communication strategies are useful when interviewing parents. Identify the purpose of each strategy listed below.

   a. Encouraging the parent to talk

   b. Directing the focus

   c. Listening and cultural awareness

   d. Silence

   e. Being empathetic

   f. Defining the problem

   g. Solving the problem

   h. Providing anticipatory guidance

   i. Avoiding blocks to communication

5. List at least three verbal strategies for conducting culturally sensitive interactions.

   a.

   b.

   c.

6. List at least three signs of information overload.

   a.

   b.

   c.

7. What considerations should the nurse be sensitive to when communicating with families through an interpreter?

8. Indicate whether the following statements regarding interpreters are true or false.

   a. T   F   Communicate directly with family members when asking questions to communicate your interest in them.

   b. T   F   Use medical terms whenever possible.

   c. T   F   Arrange to use the same interpreter in subsequent conversations with family.

   d. T   F   When a child is translating, it is important to stress literal translation of parent responses.

9. Match each communication strategy to the age group it is best used with.

   a. ____ Infants

   b. ____ Young children

   c. ____ School-age children

   d. ____ Adolescents

   1. Tell them what they will do and how they will feel.

   2. Cuddle with them.

   3. Tell them what is going on and why it is being done to them.

   4. Be attentive and do not pry.

10. Communicating with adolescents is especially challenging for the nurse. How would you establish a foundation to facilitate communication? List seven behaviors.

    a.

    b.

    c.

d.

e.

f.

g.

11. Storytelling is a communication strategy in which:
    a. the nurse listens carefully and reflects back the feelings and content of the statements to the patient.
    b. books are used in a therapeutic and supportive manner.
    c. the nurse presents statements and has the patient fill in the blanks.
    d. the nurse uses the language of the child to probe areas of his or her thinking.

12. Four nonverbal methods of communication that are used with young children are _____,

    _____, _____, and _____.

History Taking

13. List the 10 major components of a health history for the child and family.

    a.

    b.

    c.

    d.

    e.

    f.

    g.

    h.

    i.

    j.

14. What are the most important previous growth patterns to record?

    a.

    b.

    c.

    d.

Family Assessment

15. List the four structural areas of the family assessment that the nurse must consider.

    a.

    b.

    c.

    d.

16. The _____ is a very useful structural assessment tool.

17. List the four functional areas of the family assessment that the nurse must consider.

    a.

    b.

    c.

    d.

18. The Family APGAR is a screening questionnaire designed to reflect a family member's satisfaction with the functional state of the family. What does the acronym represent?

    A =

    P =

    G =

    A =

    R =

Nutritional Assessment

19. Identify the two factors that are essential in a thorough nutritional assessment.

20. A method used in the clinical examination portion of the nutritional assessment is:
    a. fundoscopy.
    b. arthroscopy.
    c. anthropometry.
    d. biopsy.

APPLYING CRITICAL THINKING TO NURSING PRACTICE

A. Interview a preschool child and his or her family.

 1. It is important to establish a setting for the interview. What is the first thing that should be said to establish this setting?

 2. Why is it important to include the parents in the problem-solving process?

 3. What blocks to communication may occur during the interview?

 4. What creative communication techniques are effective in encouraging communication with the child?

B. Mrs. Fernandez brings her daughter Susan, age 18 months, to the pediatric clinic for an annual checkup. It is the first time they have visited the clinic. Mrs. Fernandez' English is poor. The Fernandez family has been living in the United States for 6 months.

 1. List at least four verbal strategies that would enhance the cultural sensitivity of the interaction.

   a.

   b.

   c.

   d.

 2. During the interview Mrs. Fernandez focuses her comments on her other four children. How might the nurse redirect the focus of the interview?

3. What portion of the past history section of the health history is of particular importance because of the fact that Susan has been in this country only 6 months?

4. What information in the family medical history section of the health history should the nurse obtain from Mrs. Fernandez?

5. In order to assess the family home environment, you would use what two tools?

a.

b.

C. Gwen, age 8 years, was referred to the nutrition clinic by the nurse practitioner. The nurse was concerned because Gwen's weight was above the 90th percentile for her age. A complete nutritional assessment was performed.

1. Identify three methods that Gwen's mother can use to record Gwen's dietary intake.

2. Anthropometry was performed on Gwen. Why?

3. The results of the nutritional assessment revealed that Gwen's mother knows little about nutrition and that Gwen's obesity is the result of her excessive intake of nutrients. Develop two nursing diagnoses based on the assessment results.

a.

b.

Physical and Developmental Assessment of the Child

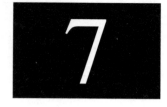

Chapter 7 provides the theoretical basis for the performance of a complete pediatric physical assessment and a developmental assessment. Since assessment is the first step in the nursing process, procedures and skills that aid in obtaining accurate and complete data are crucial to students. This chapter provides the basis for the performance of a complete physical and developmental assessment in the practice setting.

REVIEW OF ESSENTIAL CONCEPTS

General Approaches Toward Examining the Child

1. The normal sequence of examination is altered based on the child's age and developmental needs but recorded following the head-to-toe model. What five goals are accomplished by using age and development as a basis for modification of the normal sequence of examination?

    a.

    b.

    c.

    d.

    e.

2. List techniques the nurse might use with an uncooperative child.

    a.

    b.

    c.

    d.

    e.

    f.

    g.

    h.

    i.

    j.

Physical Examination

3. List the sequence of events in the physical assessment of a child.

   a.

   b.

   c.

   d.

   e.

   f.

   g.

   h.

   i.

   j.

   k.

   l.

   m.

   n.

   o.

   p.

   q.

   r.

   s.

4. In general, children whose growth patterns should be followed closely include:
   a. those whose weight falls between the 50th and 70th percentile for their age.
   b. those whose pattern of growth resembles their parents'.
   c. those who fail to show rapid weight gain in the school-age years.
   d. those who show a sudden decrease in a previously steady pattern of growth.

5. The best order for taking the vital signs in the infant is _____, _____, and

   _____.

6. Respirations in the infant are counted _____ ___ _____ _____ because they are irregular.

7. An accurate pulse in infants must be taken _____ for one full minute.

8. Match each abnormal color change with its description.

    a. ___ Cyanosis   1. Small pinpoint hemorrhages

    b. ___ Erythema   2. Blue tinge to the skin

    c. ___ Jaundice   3. Redness of the skin

    d. ___ Petechiae   4. Yellow staining of the skin

9. What should be recorded when assessing the head of an 8-month-old infant?

10. Match each term with its description.

    a. ___ Binocularity   1. One eye deviates from the point of fixation.

    b. ___ Strabismus   2. Condition indicates blindness from disuse.

    c. ___ Amblyopia   3. The patient is able to fixate on one visual field with both eyes simultaneously.

    d. ___ Cover test

                                      4. One eye is covered, and the movement of the uncovered eye is observed.

11. Criteria used when referring a 4-year-old for further evaluation of visual acuity include:
    a. 20/10 vision in both eyes on the Snellen chart.
    b. 20/40 vision in either eye on the Snellen chart.
    c. 20/30 vision in either eye on the Snellen chart.
    d. 20/60 vision in either eye on the Snellen chart.

12. Describe the normal color of the tympanic membrane.

13. T   F   Respirations in the child older than 8 years are primarily abdominal.

14. List the three normal breath sounds.

    a.

    b.

    c.

15. The two classifications of adventitious breath sounds are _____ and _____.

16. What does PMI stand for?

17. When the abdomen is auscultated, the most important finding is _____ or _____

    _____, which sound like short metallic clicks and gurgles.

18. When examining the genitalia of both males and females, the nurse notes the distribution pattern of the

    _____.

19. Define *scoliosis*.

20. T F Genu varum (bowleg) is evident when the knees are close together but the feet are spread apart.

21. Match the following cranial nerves with the portion of the cranium they control.

    a. ____ Optic nerve (II)

    b. ____ Trochlear nerve (IV)

    c. ____ Accessory nerve (XI)

    d. ____ Hypoglossal nerve (XII)

    1. Sternocleidomastoid and trapezius muscles of the shoulder

    2. Rods and cones of retina (vision)

    3. Superior oblique (SO) muscle (moves eye down and out)

    4. Muscles of the tongue

Developmental Assessment

22. T F The four major categories of the Denver II Developmental Screening Test are fine motor–adaptive, personal-social, language, gross motor.

23. T F Delays in the Denver II are defined as the failure to perform any item passed by 25% of children of the same age.

APPLYING CRITICAL THINKING TO NURSING PRACTICE

A. Tia Vang, age 3 years, is brought to the pediatric clinic for a routine physical exam. Tia has been in this country for 1 year, and Tia's father has been unable to immigrate to this country from Cambodia. Tia's immunizations are up to date. This is Tia's first visit to the clinic.

   1. Tia refuses to look at you during the health history interview. What behaviors might indicate her readiness to cooperate during the physical exam, and how might you facilitate this process?

   2. What method would you use to assess Tia's height?

3. Tia's height and weight are below the 5th percentile for children her age. What additional information should you assess before diagnosing that Tia's growth is not normal?

4. Why would you not want to take Tia's temperature orally?

5. How should Tia's vision be assessed and by what methods?

B. Perform a physical assessment on an infant and a school-age child.

1. What area do you assess after you have assessed each child's general appearance?

2. How do you obtain each child's height, and how is it recorded?

3. By what method do you obtain the heart rate in each child?

4. Data that you obtain when you assess the school-age child's behavior would include:

5. You assess the external auditory structures and visualize the internal landmarks of the ear. What did you forget to assess?

6. You evaluate the heart sounds for _____, _____, _____, and

_____.

7. The school-age child appears to have an arrhythmia. How do you determine whether this is a sinus arrhythmia?

C. Perform a developmental assessment on a toddler and a preschool child.

1. What do you tell each child's parent(s) before the test begins?

2. What information do you obtain from each child's parent(s) at the conclusion of the test?

3. How do you determine that a delay is present?

4. How do you score items on the Denver Screening Test?

5. What should you do if the results of either child's screening exam are abnormal and the mother states that the child's behavior was typical?

Health Promotion of the Newborn and Family

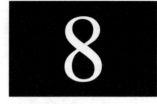

Chapter 8 introduces the factors the nurse must consider when caring for the newborn and family during delivery and the neonatal period. Profound physiologic and psychologic changes occur as the neonate adjusts to extrauterine life. Awareness of these changes enables the nurse to assess the adaptation of the neonate. At the completion of this chapter, the student will know the essential nursing care for the neonate and family. This knowledge will enable the student to assess the neonate and family and to formulate nursing goals and interventions that will promote normal physiologic and psychologic adjustment and development.

REVIEW OF ESSENTIAL CONCEPTS

Adjustment to Extrauterine Life

1. The respiratory changes that occur during the transition to extrauterine life include:

2. T F A change in the cardiovascular system that occurs after birth involves an increase in pressure in the right atrium of the heart.

3. The most important factor controlling the closure of the ductus arteriosus is:
   a. increased oxygen concentration of the blood.
   b. deposition of fibrin and cells.
   c. rise of endogenous prostaglandin.
   d. presence of metabolic acidosis.

4. Factors that predispose the neonate to heat loss include:

   a.

   b.

   c.

5. The rate of fluid exchange in the infant is _____ times greater than that of the adult. The infant's rate

   of metabolism is _____ as great as that of the adult, relative to body weight.

6. A limitation of the newborn's gastrointestinal system is:
   a. the inability to digest disaccharides.
   b. decreased transit time of food passing through the stomach and colon.
   c. increased storage of glycogen.
   d. lower esophageal sphincter pressure.

7. T F The kidney of the neonate is unable to concentrate urine.

8. Identify the three lines of defense against infection that are present in the infant.

   a.

   b.

   c.

Nursing Care of the Newborn and Family

9. The five items included in the Apgar score are:

   a.

   b.

   c.

   d.

   e.

10. The maximum score an infant can receive on the Apgar is _____.

11. Classification of infants at birth by both _____ _____ and _____

    _____ provides a more satisfactory method for predicting morbidity and mortality risks.

12. T   F   The normal head circumference of the neonate is 20 to 21 inches.

13. T   F   The normal pulse rate of the neonate is 120 to 140 beats/minute.

14. Areas to be assessed in the general appearance section of the newborn assessment include:

15. A reflex that should be present in the normal neonate is:
    a. Landau.
    b. Moro.
    c. parachute.
    d. neck-righting.

16. For the first _____ to _____ hours after birth, the infant is in the first period of reactivity.

17. Behaviors seen during the second period of reactivity include:

18. Identify an effective method of systematically assessing the infant's behavior.

19. T   F   The state of deep sleep is characterized by closed eyes, regular breathing, no movement except for sudden bodily twitches, and no eye movement.

20. Six nursing goals that are the basis for safe and effective care of the neonate are:

    a.

    b.

    c.

    d.

    e.

    f.

21. T   F   Vitamin K is administered to the newborn to prevent the occurrence of hemorrhagic disease of the newborn.

22. Why is the use of soap discouraged in the newborn period?

23. T   F   When undergoing circumcision, infants need no anesthesia since they feel no pain.

24. Cow's milk is not suitable for the infant's nutrition because it:
    a. has too few calories per ounce.
    b. has too much protein.
    c. is too dilute.
    d. has too much calcium.

25. _____ _____ is the preferred form of nutrition for all infants.

26. T   F   The process of the father's attachment to the newborn is called engrossment.

27. What are the reasons that discharge planning and care at home are of increasing importance?

APPLYING CRITICAL THINKING TO NURSING PRACTICE

A. Perform an initial and transitional assessment on a newborn based on Apgar score and periods of reactivity.

    1. The five areas you assess to determine the Apgar score include:

2. The infant received a score of 1 on the heart rate category of the Apgar. This indicates that the neonate's

   heart rate was _____.

3. The infant had little difficulty adjusting to extrauterine life. The Apgar score for this infant would be

   between _____ and _____.

4. What behaviors do you observe to indicate that the infant is in the first period of reactivity?

5. An appropriate nursing intervention in the first stage of reactivity would include:
   a. giving initial bath.
   b. administering eyedrops before child has contact with the parents.
   c. allowing mother to breast-feed.
   d. minimizing contact with parents until temperature has stabilized.

B. Determine a neonate's gestational age.

1. Why is assessment of gestational age important?

2. The six neuromuscular signs that you assess include:

3. You plot the infant's height, weight, and head circumference on standardized graphs. You determine that the infant is normal for gestational age because:

C. Perform a physical assessment on a newborn.

1. The head circumference of the infant you assess should be between _____ and _____. What should you suspect if the head circumference is significantly smaller than the chest circumference?

2. What areas do you assess when you examine the eyes of the neonate?

3. How do you determine that the infant is in the "light sleep" behavioral stage?

D. Baby Boy Florenz is a 1-day-old infant who is rooming in with his mother. Baby Florenz is a term infant who received a normal newborn examination. He is a first child.

1. Formulate at least three nursing diagnoses for Baby Florenz during the newborn period.

a.

b.

c.

2. List four nursing interventions that should be used to maintain a patent airway in Baby Florenz.

a.

b.

c.

d.

3. What is the rationale for keeping clothes and blankets loose?

4. What criteria could be used to evaluate nursing interventions aimed at maintaining a patent airway in the transition period?

5. What areas should be included in the discharge planning of Baby Florenz and his parents?

E. The Cohens have just had their first baby, Sarah. The infant received a normal newborn exam. The Cohens have been attending parenting classes in the hospital and feel comfortable about the routine care of their infant.

1. What behaviors might be assessed to determine whether the Cohens have attached to Sarah?

2. Formulate one nursing diagnosis related to the attachment process.

3. Develop six nursing interventions to facilitate the attachment process.

a.

b.

c.

d.

e.

f.

Health Problems of Newborns

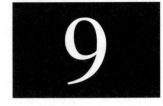

Chapter 9 is concerned with the neonate at high risk for morbidity and mortality because of conditions that are superimposed on the normal course of events associated with birth. Advances in medical technology have improved the survival rate of these compromised neonates. Students must be familiar with the complex care required by high-risk infants and their families. Effective assessment skills are paramount to successful nursing care of these infants. At the completion of this chapter, the student will be able to formulate nursing goals and interventions to provide for the normal development of the newborn and to assist the family to cope with the stress of a neonatal health problem.

REVIEW OF ESSENTIAL CONCEPTS

Birth Injuries

1. Soft-tissue injury usually occurs when there is some degree of disproportion between the

   _____ _____ and the _____ _____.

2. The most commonly observed scalp lesion is a vaguely outlined area of edematous tissue situated over the portion of the scalp that presents during a vertex delivery. Which of the following terms matches this description?
   a. caput succedaneum
   b. hydrocephalus
   c. cephalhematoma
   d. subdural hematoma

3. What bone is most commonly fractured during the birth process?

4. A neonate exhibits loss of movement on one side of the face and an absence of wrinkling of the forehead. What does this indicate?

5. Describe a chief concern in the nursing care of the neonate with brachial palsy.

Common Problems in the Newborn

6. Oral candidiasis (thrush) is an infection that commonly afflicts neonates. Are the following statements regarding candidiasis true or false?

   a. T   F   *Candida albicans* is the causative organism.

   b. T   F   The infection is characterized by white curdy patches that cannot be scraped from mucous membranes.

   c. T   F   The infection frequently follows prolonged antibiotic therapy.

   d. T   F   The infection is usually treated with systemic and local antibiotics.

7. Match each type of birthmark with its definition.

   a. ____ Capillary hemangioma

   b. ____ Port-wine stains

   c. ____ Café-au-lait spots

   d. ____ Cavernous venous
            hemangioma

   1. Involves deep vessels in the dermis, is a bluish red color, and has poorly defined margins.

   2. Multiple light brown discolorations often associated with autosomal-dominant hereditary disorders.

   3. Pink, red, or purple stains of the skin that thicken, darken, and enlarge as the child grows.

   4. Benign cutaneous tumor that involves only capillaries.

Nursing Care of the High-Risk Newborn and Family

8. The high-risk infant may be classified according to:

   a.

   b.

   c.

9. Items to be included in the gastrointestinal assessment of the infant include:

10. An accurate urinary output can be obtained by _____ diapers.

11. LBW preterm infants have difficulty with thermoregulation. The infant is kept in a heated environment to

    prevent the complication termed _____ _____.

12. Extracellular water content is _____ in a preterm infant than in a full-term infant.

13. The amount and method of feeding the preterm infant is determined by the _____ and

    _____ of the infant.

14. A major goal of care of the high-risk infant is conservation of _____.

15. Alkaline-based soaps should not be used to clean the skin of the preterm infant because they interfere with:

16. List the six categories of nursing interventions to foster development in the high-risk infant.

    a.

    b.

    c.

    d.

    e.

    f.

17. Pain assessment in the preverbal child is difficult. Assessment must be based on:

18. A pain assessment tool used in neonatal units is called NPASS, which stands for:

19. To help parents deal with the death of their infant, the nurse should allow them private time after death to:

High Risk Related to Dysmaturity

20. Match each characteristic with its corresponding type of maturity.

    a. ____ Abundant lanugo   1. Preterm

    b. ____ Presence of subcutaneous fat   2. Postmature

    c. ____ Cracked and parchment-like skin   3. Term

High Risk Related to Physiologic Factors

21. The major clinical manifestation of hyperbilirubinemia is _____.

22. Why do most newborns experience elevated bilirubin levels?

23. A common treatment for hyperbilirubinemia that involves the use of intense fluorescent light is called

    _____.

24. Major causes of increased erythrocyte destruction are _____ and _____ incompatibility, which result in hemolytic disease of the newborn.

25. The primary aim of therapeutic management of alloimmunization (hemolytic disease of newborns) is

    _____ by administering _____.

26. A factor in the pathophysiology of respiratory distress syndrome is:
    a. decreased pulmonary vascular resistance.
    b. increase in pulmonary blood flow.
    c. deficient production of surfactant.
    d. respiratory alkalosis.

27. The most serious cardiovascular disorders of the newborn are the _____ _____ defects.

28. List the causes of neonatal seizures.

    a.

    b.

    c.

    d.

    e.

    f.

    g.

High Risk Related to Infectious Processes

29. T   F   The diagnosis of sepsis is made on the basis of blood, urine, and CSF cultures.

30. Three factors play an important role in the development of NEC; they are:

31. Clinical manifestations specific to NEC include:

High Risk Related to Maternal Conditions

32. A characteristic clinical manifestation of the infant of a mother whose diabetes is not under complete control is:
    a. hyperglycemia.
    b. loss of subcutaneous fat.
    c. absence of vernix caseosa.
    d. large for gestational age.

33. List appropriate drug therapies to decrease withdrawal side effects for narcotic-addicted infants.

Congenital Abnormalities

34. A test to detect maternal infection that may be teratogenic is called TORCHS. Explain this acronym.

35. A recognized pattern of congenital malformations due to a single specific cause is called a

    _____.

36. List some of the most recognized teratogenic drugs (chemical agents).

37. _____ are inherited diseases caused by the absence or deficiency of a substance essential to cellular metabolism, usually an enzyme.

Inborn Errors of Metabolism

38. T   F   Phenylketonuria (PKU) is inherited as an autosomal-recessive trait.

39. The hepatic enzyme, _____ _____, is absent in PKU.

40. What is the most effective method of identifying neonates with PKU?

41. T   F   Infants with galactosemia usually display notable abnormalities at birth.

APPLYING CRITICAL THINKING TO NURSING PRACTICE

A. Baby Boy Jacobs is admitted to the newborn nursery following an uncomplicated vertex delivery. During the initial assessment it is noted that he has a caput succedaneum over the right frontal area.

   1. Differentiate between the following types of head trauma that can occur during the birth process.

     a. Caput succedaneum

     b. Cephalhematoma

   2. Identify the two major nursing goals associated with the care of the neonate with birth-related head trauma.

     a.

     b.

B. Care for a high-risk infant.

   1. What is the best method to use in classifying the high-risk infant?

   2. Why is the prevention of infection such an important goal for the high-risk infant?

   3. What nursing diagnosis addresses the nursing goal "Will receive nourishment and exhibit appropriate weight gain"?

   4. What assessment parameter can you use to determine whether the infant is getting adequate nutrition?

5. How do you evaluate whether the interventions are successful in preventing skin breakdown?

6. Four nursing goals developed to prevent an alteration in family process are:

   a.

   b.

   c.

   d.

7. What is the rationale for encouraging the parents to visit the infant?

C. Care for a neonate who is receiving phototherapy.

   1. What two factors are primarily responsible for the development of physiologic jaundice in the newborn?

      a.

      b.

   2. When would the nurse expect the following phases of physiologic jaundice to occur in the full-term infant?

      a. Onset

      b. Peak

      c. Resolution

   3. Identify the nursing interventions associated with the care of the child receiving phototherapy.

      a.

      b.

      c.

      d.

      e.

D. Cindy is a premature infant in the ICU. She has recovered from her respiratory distress and has been diagnosed as having an intraventricular hemorrhage. She is suspected of having sepsis.

   1. Postnatally, how might Cindy have obtained her infection?

   2. What are some of the findings that can be observed that suggest sepsis?

   3. The most important nursing goal for Cindy is:

E. Michael is a premature infant who experienced severe intestinal ischemia at birth. Oral feedings were started within the first 24 hours. He is now having problems with feedings. Necrotizing enterocolitis (NEC) is suspected. He is also anemic.

   1. What factor in Michael's history predisposes him to the development of NEC?

   2. The most important nursing responsibility when caring for infants who are at risk for developing NEC is

   _____ _____.

   3. Nonspecific clinical signs that would alert the nurse to the presence of NEC include:

F. Terry is a 3-day-old infant born to a mother who developed diabetes during pregnancy. Terry was admitted to ICU for observation.

   1. Why is hypoglycemia a common occurrence in infants of mothers with diabetes?

   2. Why is feeding begun so early with these infants?

3. Nursing responsibilities for the very large infant of a mother with diabetes include monitoring the infant for signs of birth injuries such as:

   a.

   b.

   c.

Health Promotion of the Infant and Family

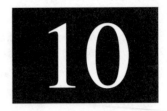

Chapter 10 explores infancy, the period from birth to 12 months of age. Infancy is the period of the fastest gain in physical size and of the most dramatic developmental achievements of the entire life span. It is characterized by an orderly progression of physical, cognitive, and social maturation, which is affected by both positive and negative influences. Upon completion of this chapter, the student will have the necessary information base to counsel parents on optimal development.

REVIEW OF ESSENTIAL CONCEPTS

Promoting Optimum Growth and Development

1. An infant who is 5 months of age should have _____ his or her birth weight.

2. A physiologic characteristic of a 5-month-old is:
   a. the presence of iron deficiency anemia.
   b. mature kidney function.
   c. eruption of the first tooth.
   d. adult level of fat absorption.

3. List two reasons why infants are susceptible to dehydration.

   a.

   b.

4. By what age should binocularity be well established?

5. The fine motor development of a normal 3-month-old can best be described as:
   a. the ability to transfer objects.
   b. the ability to actively hold a rattle (but will not reach for it).
   c. the ability to voluntarily grasp an object.
   d. the presence of a pincer grasp.

6. The gross motor development of a normal 6-month-old can best be described as:
   a. the ability to roll from back to abdomen.
   b. the ability to sit unsupported.
   c. the ability to crawl.
   d. the ability to pull self to standing position.

7. T   F   The infant is in Erikson's stage of developing a sense of trust.

8. The infant is in Piaget's stage of _____ and then _____ circular reactions.

9. The two components of cognitive development that are necessary for attachment are:

    a.

    b.

10. T   F   At 3 months, the infant displays a definite preference for the mother.

11. *Stranger anxiety* is defined as:

12. Infants can comprehend the meaning of the word *no* by the age of _____ or _____ months.

13. Stimulation (in the form of play) is as important for _____ growth as food is for biologic growth.

14. Appropriate toys for a 4-month-old child are:

15. T   F   Problems with dental development are associated with the use of a pacifier.

16. A quick guide to assessment of deciduous teeth during the first year is:

17. The main reason for shoes when the child has started walking is for _____.

Promoting Optimum Health During Infancy

18. Human milk is deficient in the mineral _____ and should be given after 6 months of age.

19. T   F   The amount of formula that a 6-month-old should be taking at each of five feedings is 8 ounces.

20. List the reasons why it is not advisable to introduce solid foods to a 3-month-old infant.

    a.

    b.

    c.

21. Identify and offer a rationale for the first solid introduced into the infant's diet.

22. T F   Each new solid food is introduced alone for 4 to 7 days to detect food allergies.

23. The management of night crying includes:
    a. putting the child in his or her own bed while the child is awake.
    b. arranging a sleeping area with brothers or sisters.
    c. placing the child in the parents' bed for comfort.
    d. rocking the child until he or she is asleep.

24. T F   During infancy, toothpaste can be used to clean erupting teeth.

25. Common reactions to a DTP immunization include:

26. What is the leading cause of fatal injury in children under 1 year of age?

27. What is the leading cause of fatal injury in children older than 1 year of age?

APPLYING CRITICAL THINKING TO NURSING PRACTICE

A. Mrs. Backer brings 7-month-old Jerry to the well-child clinic for his checkup. During the course of the examination Mrs. Backer says that Jerry is teething, has shown little interest in breast-feeding, and cries when she leaves the room. She has been reading *Parents* magazine and is concerned that Jerry is not "doing" what the magazine states he should be "doing."

   1. Jerry was 7 pounds at birth. At this visit he weighs 16 pounds. Is this weight normal for his age?

   2. What fine motor, gross motor, language, and social developmental milestones does the nurse assess in Jerry that lead to a determination that Jerry is developing normally?

   3. What nursing intervention might you suggest to Mrs. Backer regarding Jerry's crying when she leaves the room?

4. List the interventions that Mrs. Backer could implement to relieve teething pain.

a.

b.

5. What might Jerry's lack of interest in breast-feeding indicate, and what intervention should you suggest to Jerry's mother?

6. List the interventions that Mrs. Backer can use to promote good dental health in Jerry.

a.

b.

c.

d.

B. Rachel is a 4-month-old infant who is at the clinic for her checkup. Rachel's mother states that she is having difficulty managing Rachel because nothing she tries works twice, and she is concerned about Rachel's sleeping pattern.

1. What behaviors are assessed to determine whether Rachel is in Piaget's stage of secondary circular reactions?

2. What should the nurse assess regarding Rachel's sleeping pattern?

a.

b.

c.

d.

e.

3. Rachel's mother will start Rachel on solid foods before the next checkup. What guidelines should be given to her?

a.

b.

c.

d.

e.

f.

g.

C. Administer immunizations to an infant.

1. What two nursing interventions should be used to properly store immunizations?

a.

b.

2. What is the safest site for administration of immunizations in the infant?

D. Teach the parents of an infant who is 8 to 12 months old how to prevent accidental injury to their child.

1. What developmental landmarks do you assess in the infant that predispose him or her to injury?

2. What interventions might you suggest to prevent burns in the child?

a.

b.

c.

d.

e.

3. What is the rationale for keeping the bathroom door closed?

4. Why is choking still such a problem in this age group?

5. What is the rationale for not administering medications as candy?

6. The parents inform you that their infant frequently spends time at the grandparents' home. What nursing intervention should you suggest to them?

Health Problems of Infants

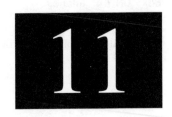

Chapter 11 introduces common health problems of the first year of life. They are usually influenced by environmental factors affecting the physical or psychologic development of the child because of the infant's immature physiologic system. Students need to be aware of these health problems because prompt identification and treatment will avert problems later in life. At the completion of this chapter, the student will be able to provide nursing care to infants with these health problems and their families.

REVIEW OF ESSENTIAL CONCEPTS

Nutritional Disturbances

1. Vitamin A deficiency correlates with _____ (increased, decreased) morbidity and mortality in children with measles.

2. Toxic reactions can be caused by overdose of vitamins. An excessive dose is defined as:

3. What vitamin supplement to prevent neural tube birth defects is recommended for all women of childbearing age? What is the daily recommended dose?

4. The deficiency of vitamin C is referred to as:
   a. rickets.
   b. scurvy.
   c. pellagra.
   d. beriberi.

5. T   F   Vitamin D is necessary for the absorption of calcium and phosphorus in the body.

6. The clinical manifestations of a zinc deficiency include:

7. Which type of vegetarian diet poses the least risk for deficiencies in the infant diet?

8. What are the major deficiencies in the stricter vegetarian diets?

9. What has replaced the traditional Basic Four Food Groups?

10. The American Academy of Pediatrics recommends that fat intake for children over 2 years of age should

    provide no more than _____ percent of calories.

11. Malnutrition is a major health problem in the world in children under 5 years of age. What are the two major causes of this problem?

    a.

    b.

12. *Kwashiorkor* is defined as:
    a. deficiency of calories.
    b. deficiency of calories and protein.
    c. deficiency of fats and carbohydrates.
    d. deficiency of protein with adequate calories.

13. Food sensitivities are divided into two categories. List the categories, and identify the primary cause of reactions in each of the categories.

    a.

    b.

14. Define the term *atopy*.

15. What is the most definitive method of diagnosing cow's milk intolerance?

16. Lactose intolerance involves deficiency of the enzyme _____.

17. Manifestations of lactose intolerance are:

Feeding Difficulties

18. Match each feeding problem with its definition.

    a. ____   Regurgitation   1. Paroxysmal abdominal pain

    b. ____   Spitting up   2. Return of undigested food from the stomach

    c. ____   Colic   3. Dribbling of unswallowed formula

19. List the elements of the nursing assessment that would be noted regarding colic.

    a.

    b.

    c.

    d.

    e.

    f.

    g.

    h.

    i.

20. T   F   A characteristic of children with nonorganic failure to thrive is their intense interest in social inter-
            action.

21. Parents of the failure-to-thrive infant are at increased risk for attachment problems because of:

    a.

    b.

    c.

22. What is the most important goal of therapeutic management of the failure-to-thrive infant?

23. List the guidelines that should be used for the feeding of the nonorganic failure-to-thrive infant.

    a.

    b.

    c.

d.

e.

f.

g.

h.

i.

Disorders of Unknown Etiology

24. In order to prevent SIDS, the American Academy of Pediatrics recommends that healthy infants be placed in

the _____ (supine, prone) position to sleep.

25. Flattening of the occipital skull is called _____ _____.

26. One of the most important aspects of the care of the parents following a SIDS death is:

27. ALTE is an acronymn for _____ _____-_____ _____.

28. The most widely used test in the diagnostic evaluation of apnea of infancy is the

_____.

29. The therapeutic management of the infant with apnea involves the use of:

30. Three safety measures that the nurse should discuss with parents of an infant being monitored at home are:

a.

b.

c.

| **APPLYING CRITICAL THINKING TO NURSING PRACTICE** |

A. Mr. Morrison brings his 10-month-old son into the pediatric clinic for a well-child visit. Upon examination it is noted that the child's weight gain has leveled off, and he exhibits signs of a niacin deficiency. The Morrisons belong to the Seventh Day Adventist faith and are vegetarians.

   1. What risk factors should the nurse have assessed in previous well-child visits that might have prevented the nutritional problems?

   2. It is important during the nutritional assessment of the Morrison's infant that the nurse assess:

   3. List the items that would be included as interventions to help alleviate the nutritional problems of the Morrison's infant.

      a.

      b.

      c.

      d.

      e.

   4. How would you evaluate whether your interventions were successful in treating the nutritional problem?

B. Care for a child who has nonorganic failure to thrive (FTT) and the child's family.

   1. List four primary nursing goals in the nutritional management of FTT.

      a.

      b.

      c.

      d.

2. To evaluate whether the interventions have been successful in alleviating the nutritional problem, you would evaluate whether:

a.

b.

c.

C. Mr. and Mrs. Cohen arrive in the emergency room with their infant. The Cohens discovered that their infant had stopped breathing and called the rescue team, but the child could not be resuscitated.

1. List the interventions that should be used to support the parents.

a.

b.

c.

d.

2. What intervention could be used to help the parents adjust to the loss?

a.

b.

c.

D. Tommy, a 1-month-old infant, is admitted to the hospital for a diagnostic workup for apnea of infancy. Tommy's parents called the pediatrician when they noticed that there were periods where he stopped breathing and turned "blue."

1. Why is safety a major area of nursing intervention if the infant is to be monitored at home?

2. What is the rationale for informing the local utility company and rescue squad of the home monitoring?

3. It must be stressed that monitors are only effective if they are _____ and there is a

_____ to alarms.

Health Promotion of the Toddler and Family

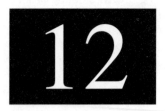

Chapter 12 presents the issues relevant to the toddler period of development, which is a time of accelerated psychosocial, cognitive, and adaptive changes. At the completion of this chapter, the student will understand the toddler's growth and development needs and areas of special concern to parents. This knowledge enables the student to develop nursing goals and interventions that provide support for the normal development of the toddler and help the parents cope with the associated developmental difficulties.

REVIEW OF ESSENTIAL CONCEPTS

Promoting Optimum Growth and Development

1. The toddler period is the time between _____ and _____ of age.

2. The growth rate slows considerably during the toddler years, and the birth weight is quadrupled by

   _____ years of age.

3. T   F   When plotted on height and weight graphs, the toddler's growth curve is usually a steady, upward curve, which is steplike in nature.

4. Why does the toddler exhibit a squat, potbellied appearance?

5. Visual acuity of _____ is considered acceptable during the toddler years.

6. One of the most prominent changes in the gastrointestinal system during the toddler period is the voluntary

   control of _____.

7. What is the major gross motor skill acquired during the toddler years?

8. Identify the seven major psychosocial developmental tasks that must be dealt with during the toddler years.

   a.

   b.

   c.

   d.

e.

f.

g.

9. According to Erikson, the developmental task of toddlerhood is acquiring a sense of

_____ while overcoming a sense of _____ and _____.

10. Identify two characteristics that are typical of toddlers in their quest for autonomy.

a.

b.

11. According to Erikson, the development of ego is evident when the child is able to:

12. A child of 21 months would be expected to be in Piaget's stage of:
    a. tertiary circular reactions.
    b. preoperations.
    c. coordination of secondary schemata and their application to new situations.
    d. secondary circular reactions.
    e. invention of new means through mental combinations.

13. Identify the level of cognitive development the child enters at approximately 2 years of age.

14. A toddler's reasoning can best be described as being:
    a. transductive.
    b. inductive.
    c. deductive.

15. Match each term related to toddler behavior with its definition.

a. ____ Transductive reasoning	1. The need to maintain sameness and reliability.
b. ____ Centration	2. Thinking that progresses from the particular to the particular.
c. ____ Ritualism	3. The tendency to focus on one aspect rather than considering all possible alternatives.
d. ____ Animism	
e. ____ Negativism	4. Persistent negative response to requests.
	5. Attribution of lifelike qualities to inanimate objects.

16. T   F   The development of body image closely parallels cognitive development.

17. Briefly describe the two phases of the toddler's task of differentiation of self from significant others.

   a. Separation

   b. Individuation

18. T   F   The most striking feature of language development in the toddler is the number of new vocabulary words acquired.

19. The typical child of 2 years has a vocabulary of approximately _____ words, and approximately

   _____ percent of this speech is understandable.

20. The toddler's developing skill of _____ influences all areas of personal-social behavior.

21. The solitary play of infancy progresses to _____ play in the toddler.

22. The child of 2 years can be expected to:
   a. use expressive jargon.
   b. build a tower of 8 cubes.
   c. have a vocabulary of 500 words.
   d. run fairly well with a wide stance.

23. By age 30 months, the child's birth weight is _____.

24. Physical and psychological readiness for toilet training is not completed until approximately _____ to

   _____ months.

25. T   F   Bowel training is usually accomplished before bladder training in the toddler.

26. Sibling rivalry seems to be most pronounced in the _____ child.

27. T   F   It is advisable to prepare the toddler for the birth of a sibling at least 6 months in advance.

28. To minimize sibling rivalry, the parents should _____ the toddler in caregiving activities.

29. Temper tantrums are a means by which toddlers assert their _____.

30. One method by which a parent can deal with negativism is by reducing:

Promoting Optimum Health During Toddlerhood

31. The decreased nutritional requirements of the toddler are manifested in a phenomenon known as

    _____ _____.

32. A good rule of thumb in determining the appropriate serving size for a toddler is to give _____

    _____ of food for each year of age.

33. The most effective methods for plaque removal are _____ and _____.

34. When adequate amounts of _____ are ingested, the incidence of tooth decay is

    _____.

35. T   F   Sugars, especially sucrose, are highly cariogenic.

36. Which of the following statements accurately describes nursing-bottle caries?
    a. Nursing-bottle caries occur in children between 8 and 18 months of age.
    b. The syndrome is distinguished by protruding upper front teeth resulting from sucking on a hard nipple.
    c. The syndrome does not occur when the child has been previously breast-fed.
    d. Giving a bottle of milk at naptime or bedtime predisposes the child to this syndrome.

37. _____ cause more deaths in children 4 years of age or younger than in any other childhood
    period except adolescence.

38. What is the implication of the previous statement?

39. The convertible restraint car seat is switched to the forward-facing position when the child weighs _____

    pounds and is _____ year(s) of age.

40. Children can be switched to regular seat belt restraints when they weigh _____ pounds or are

    _____ year(s) old.

41. _____ are the most common type of thermal injury in children.

42. The major reason for accidental poisoning in young children is:

| **APPLYING CRITICAL THINKING TO NURSING PRACTICE** |

A. A young mother brings her 2-year-old son, David, into a well-child clinic for a routine checkup. The child is apprehensive and clings to his mother. Height and weight are obtained; the child's height is 35 in (89 cm), and his weight is 30 lb (13.64 kg).

1. Plot David's height and weight on a growth chart. How do his measurements compare with norms for this age?

   a. Height

   b. Weight

2. David's mother is concerned because he has gained only 2 pounds and grown 2 inches since his 18-month checkup. What information should be provided to his mother regarding toddler growth patterns?

3. Identify three developmental milestones that David should have accomplished in the following areas.

   a. Gross motor development

   b. Fine motor development

   c. Language development

4. David's mother states that when he is with other children of his age, he plays near them but makes no attempt to interact with them. What information regarding the toddler's play habits should be provided?

5. What information should be provided to David's mother regarding the selection of appropriate play activities?

   a.

   b.

6. David is not yet toilet-trained. His mother asks when she should begin trying to train him. The nurse's most appropriate response should be:

   a. David will need to be able to sit on the toilet for 10 to 15 minutes at a time.

   b. A factor in successful training is the child's desire to please the mother by controlling impulses to defecate and urinate.

   c. Bladder training should be attempted first since the child usually has a stronger and more regular urge to urinate.

   d. Attempts to begin toilet training before age 3 are usually unsuccessful because myelinization of the spinal cord is incomplete.

7. David's mother asks questions about dental care. List four components for a preventive dental hygiene teaching plan for a toddler.

   a.

   b.

   c.

   d.

B. Interview the parents of a toddler about negativism, management of temper tantrums, and eating and sleep patterns. Answer the following questions and include specific responses that illustrate these concepts.

   1. How is negativism most often manifested in the toddler?

   2. The most effective method of dealing with negativism is to reduce the opportunity for a

      _____ _____.

   3. How does negativism contribute to the toddler's acquisition of a sense of autonomy?

   4. Why are temper tantrums so prevalent in the toddler age group?

   5. Why does physiologic anorexia occur in the toddler?

6. Identify four eating behaviors that are characteristic of the toddler.

   a.

   b.

   c.

   d.

7. Why is nutritional counseling for parents with toddlers an important nursing intervention?

8. Sleep problems are common in this age group. The problems are probably related to:

9. What are two interventions a parent can use to reduce sleep problems?

   a.

   b.

C. Assess the home of a toddler for the presence of potential safety hazards. Answer the following questions, and include specific examples that illustrate these concepts.

   1. Identify the two key determinants in injury prevention.

      a.

      b.

   2. Why is there a critical increase in injuries during the toddler years?

   3. What categories of injuries are common during the toddler years?

      a.

      b.

      c.

      d.

      e.

f.

g.

4. Identify at least five factors in the home that could pose a safety hazard to the toddler.

    a.

    b.

    c.

    d.

    e.

5. Match the following developmental accomplishments with the appropriate safety measures. Answers may be used more than once.

    a. ___ Walks, runs, climbs   1. Closely supervise when near a source of water.

    b. ___ Exhibits curiosity   2. Choose toys without removable parts.

    c. ___ Pulls objects   3. Turn pot handles toward back of stove.

    d. ___ Puts things in mouth   4. Place all toxic agents out of reach in a locked cabinet.

                                            5. Place child-protector caps on all medicines and poisons.

                                            6. Cover electrical outlets with protective plastic caps.

                                            7. Avoid giving sharp or pointed objects.

                                            8. Keep tablecloth out of child's reach.

                                            9. Lock fences and doors if children are not directly supervised.

6. What causes more accidental deaths after the age of 1 year than any other type of injury? What intervention can parents employ to reduce the majority of injuries?

Health Promotion of the Preschooler and Family

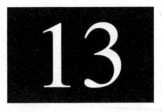

Chapter 13 focuses on the development of the child in the preschool period, which spans the ages of 3 to 5 years. During this period the child completes what is considered to be the most critical period of emotional and psychologic development. Upon completion of the chapter, the student will have a knowledge of the preschooler's needs and be aware of the areas that are of special concern to parents. This knowledge will enable the student to develop nursing goals and interventions that provide support for the normal development of the preschooler and assist parents in coping with the associated developmental difficulties.

REVIEW OF ESSENTIAL CONCEPTS

Promoting Optimum Growth and Development

1. The preschool years, a period from _____ years of age to the completion of the _____ year, comprise the end of early childhood.

2. During the preschool years, physical growth continues to _____ and _____.

3. T   F   Most bodily systems of the preschooler are mature and stable and can adjust to moderate stress and change.

4. According to Erikson, the chief psychosocial task of the preschool period is acquiring a sense of

   _____.

5. A major task for preschoolers is the development of the _____, or conscience.

6. One of the tasks related to the preschool period is _____ for school and scholastic learning.

7. The two stages of Piaget's preoperational phase are:

   a.

   b.

8. Identify one of the major transitions that occurs during the preoperational stage of development.

9. _____ remains primarily a vehicle of egocentric communication.

10. Define the term *causality*.

11. Preschoolers' thinking is often described as _____, since they believe that their thoughts are all-powerful.

12. T   F   Preschoolers have poorly defined body boundaries and little knowledge of their internal anatomy.

13. List two examples that demonstrate that the preschool child has relinquished much of the stranger anxiety and fear of separation of earlier years.

    a.

    b.

14. T   F   During the preschool years, vocabulary increases dramatically.

15. The typical child of 5 years can be expected to have a vocabulary consisting of at least _____ words.

16. Preschoolers form 3- and 4-word sentences and include only the most essential words to convey a meaning.

    Such speech is termed _____.

17. How does the preschooler differ from the toddler in demonstrating a sense of autonomy?

    a.

    b.

18. The type of play that is most apparent during the preschool years is _____ play.

19. The appearance of imaginary playmates usually occurs between the ages of _____ and _____ years.

20. Identify three functions that imaginary playmates serve.

    a.

    b.

    c.

21. The child of 4 years of age can be expected to:
    a. walk down stairs using alternate footing.
    b. tie shoelaces.
    c. use sentences of 6 to 8 words.
    d. question what parents think.

22. List three opportunities that nursery schools and daycare centers provide for children.

    a.

    b.

    c.

23. What factors should parents consider when choosing a preschool or daycare program?

    a.

    b.

    c.

    d.

    e.

    f.

    g.

    h.

    i.

    j.

24. In terms of overall evaluation of a program, the most important factor is _____

    _____ of the facility.

25. List the two rules that govern answering a child's questions about sex or other sensitive issues.

    a.

    b.

26. _____ in the preschool child is a normal part of sexual curiosity and exploration.

27. Identify some of the child's most common fears during the preschool years.

    a.

    b.

    c.

    d.

    e.

    f.

28. Define the term *aggression*.

29. The differences between "normal" aggression and "problematic" aggression are:

   a.

   b.

   c.

   d.

   e.

30. The most critical period for speech development occurs between _____ and _____ years of age.

31. Why is stuttering a common occurrence during the preschool years?

32. T   F   The Denver Articulation Screening Examination is an excellent tool to assess articulation skills in the child.

Promoting Optimum Health During the Preschool Years

33. T   F   Nutritional requirements for preschoolers are similar to those for toddlers.

34. In children over 2 years of age, intake of fiber, fruits, and vegetables should equal the child's age plus

   _____ in grams/day.

35. _____ years of age is a period for the resurgence of finicky eating.

36. What fact should be stressed to parents of preschoolers in the course of nutritional counseling?

37. T   F   Parental interventions to help the child deal with nightmares and sleep terrors are the same.

38. Why is dental care essential for the preschool child?

   a.

   b.

39. T   F   During the preschool years, the emphasis on injury prevention is placed on education for safety and potential hazards to prevent injury.

> **APPLYING CRITICAL THINKING TO NURSING PRACTICE**

A. Frank Squire, who will be 5 years old next month, is brought to the pediatrician's office by his mother for a well-child visit. Height and weight are obtained. The child's height is 42 in (106.6 cm), and his weight is 39 lb (17.69 kg).

1. Plot Frank's height and weight on a growth chart. How do his measurements compare with the norms for this age?

   a. Height

   b. Weight

2. What information could be given to Frank's mother regarding the physical growth of the preschooler?

3. Before the physical examination, the nurse questions Mrs. Squire about Frank's developmental progress. Identify three developmental milestones that Frank should have accomplished in the following areas.

   a. Gross motor development

   b. Fine motor development

   c. Language development

4. Mrs. Squire says that Frank spends most of his time playing with his imaginary friend, Oscar. She wonders whether this phase will pass. What information should be given to her?

5. Mrs. Squire states that Frank has several toys but only plays with a few. What types of playthings and activities could be recommended to foster Frank's development?

    a. Physical play

    b. Dramatic play

6. Mrs. Squire is very concerned about child safety. What developmental achievements make Frank more prone to injury?

B. Interview the parents of a child who attends a preschool program. Answer the following questions and include specific responses to illustrate these concepts.

    1. What is the most important aspect of a preschool or daycare program?

    2. What should parents do when visiting a facility they are considering for their child?

       a.

       b.

       c.

       d.

    3. How should parents prepare the child for the preschool experience?

       a.

       b.

       c.

       d.

C. Interview the parents of a preschool child about the following common parental concerns: sex education, sleep disturbances, and eating patterns. Answer the following questions and include specific responses to illustrate these concepts.

1. Why is the preschool stage of development appropriate for beginning sex education?

2. Identify the rationales for each of the following interventions that promote the sex education of the preschool child.

   a. Determining what the child thinks

   b. Being honest

3. What sleep problems occur in this age group that might concern parents?

4. What interventions could be suggested to parents to deal with nightmares?

   a.

   b.

   c.

   d.

5. Health problems as an adult can be influenced by eating patterns established in the preschool years. What goal would you encourage parents to achieve related to the intake of fat in this age group?

6. What is the primary concern of parents regarding the preschool child's diet?

7. Describe one intervention that might decrease this parental concern.

Health Problems of Toddlers and Preschoolers

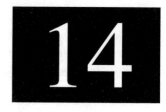

Chapter 14 introduces nursing considerations essential to the care of the young child experiencing health problems that have the potential for long-term consequences if appropriate interventions are not instituted promptly. At the completion of this chapter, the student will have a knowledge of the commonly encountered health problems of early childhood. This knowledge will enable the student to develop nursing goals and interventions directed at returning the child and the family to a state of optimum health.

REVIEW OF ESSENTIAL CONCEPTS

Infectious Disorders

1. Identify four factors that are helpful in identifying communicable diseases in children.

    a.

    b.

    c.

    d.

2. List four nursing goals in the care of the child and family with a communicable disease.

    a.

    b.

    c.

    d.

3. Prevention of communicable disease consists of two components. Identify them.

    a.

    b.

4. The most important procedure to use to prevent the spread of infection is _____.

5. List the three groups of children who are at risk for developing serious or fatal complications from communicable diseases.

    a.

    b.

    c.

6. Varicella-zoster virus (VZV) causes two diseases; they are _____ (_____ _____)

   and _____ _____ (_____).

7. What drug reduces the morbidity and mortality of children with measles?

8. List some measures to relieve the itching skin rashes caused by a communicable disease.

   a.

   b.

   c.

   d.

   e.

9. Match each communicable disease with its etiologic agent.

   a. ____ Diphtheria   1. Paramyxovirus

   b. ____ Mumps   2. Human parvovirus B19 (HPV)

   c. ____ Erythema infectiosum   3. *Corynebacterium diphtheriae*
           (fifth disease)
                                          4. *Bordetella pertussis*
   d. ____ Pertussis
           (whooping cough)   5. Group A β–hemolytic streptococci

   e. ____ Scarlet fever

10. Define *conjunctivitis*.

11. Identify the most common causes of conjunctivitis in the following groups.

    a. Recurrent conjunctivitis in infants

    b. Acute conjunctivitis in children

12. Bacterial conjunctivitis is usually treated with:
    a. corticosteroids.
    b. topical antibacterial agents.
    c. oral antibiotics.

13. The two major nursing goals in the care of the child with conjunctivitis are:

    a.

    b.

14. An important nursing consideration regarding spread of bacterial conjunctivitis is:

15. What are the two types of stomatitis typically seen in children?

    a.

    b.

16. Differentiate between aphthous and herpetic stomatitis by labeling the following clinical characteristics appropriately.

    a. ____ A benign but painful condition whose cause
    is unknown

    b. ____ Caused by the herpes simplex virus (HSV)

    c. ____ Small, whitish ulcerations surrounded by
    red border

    d. ____ Commonly called "cold sores" or "fever
    blisters"

    1. Aphthous stomatitis

    2. Herpetic gingivostomatitis

Intestinal Parasitic Diseases

17. The two most common parasitic infections among children in the United States are

    _____ and _____.

18. Nursing responsibilities related to parasitic intestinal infections are directed toward:

    a.

    b.

    c.

19. The nurse's most important function in relation to parasitic infections is:

20. _____ _____ is the most common intestinal parasitic pathogen in the United States.

21. _____, or _____, is the most common helminthic infection in the United States.

22. T   F   The principal symptom of pinworms is intense perianal itching.

23. List six symptoms that might indicate the presence of perianal itching caused by pinworms in a young child who has difficulty verbalizing.

   a.

   b.

   c.

   d.

   e.

   f.

24. What is the most common test for diagnosing pinworms?

Ingestion of Injurious Agents

25. Briefly describe the Poison Prevention Packaging Act of 1970.

26. Identify the developmental characteristics of young children that predispose them to poisoning by ingestion.

   a.

   b.

   c.

   d.

27. List the three principles of emergency treatment following the ingestion of toxic agents.

   a.

   b.

   c.

28. One method of inducing vomiting at home is through the administration of _____

   _____, which should be administered only with the advice of the Poison Control Center.

29. Identify the indications for gastric lavage.

    a.

    b.

    c.

30. T   F   Vomiting is indicated in the treatment of an ingested corrosive substance.

31. T   F   Ingestion of plant parts is one of the most common causes of childhood poisoning.

32. The immediate danger from most hydrocarbons is _____.

33. An antidote to acetaminophen poisoning is _____.

34. Initial treatment of acute salicylate poisoning is:

35. Young children are at risk for lead poisoning because:

36. The most frequent source of acute childhood lead poisoning is deteriorating _____-_____

    _____ in older homes or lead-contaminated _____ in the yard.

37. The most serious and irreversible side effects of lead intoxication are those that affect the _____ system.

38. T   F   Erythrocyte protoporphyrin (EP) level is a sensitive indicator of low lead exposure and is used routinely as a screening test.

39. Diagnosis of lead poisoning is made by measuring blood lead levels. The blood lead level determines

    _____ _____.

40. List three commonly used chelating drugs.

    a.

    b.

    c.

41. The most important nursing goal (and other professionals' goal) related to lead poisoning is:

Child Maltreatment

42. _____ _____ is a broad term that includes intentional physical abuse or neglect, emotional abuse or neglect, and sexual abuse of children.

43. Define the term *Munchausen Syndrome by Proxy (MSP)*.

44. What three broad factors seem to predispose children to physical abuse?

    a.

    b.

    c.

45. Abusive parents who report that they were _____ _____ as children are

    _____ (more, less) likely to injure their own children.

46. List six types of sexual abuse.

    a.

    b.

    c.

    d.

    e.

    f.

47. Identify the four broad nursing goals associated with child maltreatment.

    a.

    b.

    c.

    d.

APPLYING CRITICAL THINKING TO NURSING PRACTICE

A. Mrs. Braun brings her 4-year-old daughter, Jill, to the pediatric clinic. She tells the nurse practitioner that Jill has been scratching herself around the anus and has been sleeping restlessly. A tentative diagnosis of pinworm infection is made.

1. How would a diagnosis of pinworms be confirmed?

2. Identify three nursing goals associated with pinworm infection in a child.

   a.

   b.

   c.

B. Spend a day in a hospital emergency room to observe the types of poisoning that occur and their emergency treatment. Answer the following questions and include specific examples to illustrate these concepts.

1. Identify at least three nursing interventions for each of the following areas of emergency treatment.

   a. Assessment

   b. Gastric decontamination

   c. Prevention of recurrence

2. Salicylates and acetaminophen are the two most commonly ingested drugs among children. For each of the following statements regarding ingestion, mark "A" if the statement applies to acetaminophen ingestion and "S" if it applies to salicylate ingestion.

   a. _____ Hyperpnea and hyperpyrexia are common clinical manifestations.

   b. _____ In chronic overdose, it can cause bleeding tendencies.

   c. _____ Bleeding is treated by vitamin K.

   d. _____ Acute overdose results in hepatic damage.

C. Assess a specific child's environment with regard to its potential for lead poisoning. Answer the following questions and include specific examples that illustrate these concepts.

1. What early signs of low-dose-exposure lead poisoning and its effect on the nervous system should the nurse be alert to when performing an assessment?

2. If, during the assessment, the presence of lead poisoning is suspected, what should the nurse's initial goal be?

3. Blood lead level determines the type of intervention for the child with lead poisoning. At what level does the child require each of the following?

   a. Clinical management, environmental evaluation, and lead hazard control: _____ μg/dl

   b. Chelation therapy: _____ μg/dl

   c. Immediate medical treatment and chelation therapy: _____ μg/dl

4. What are the nursing interventions for the following nursing goals regarding chelation therapy?

   a. Pain control

   b. Prevent fibrotic tissue

   c. Prevent complications with kidneys and of seizures

5. Since lead poisoning can occur in children from all socioeconomic strata, what factors regarding food preparation and diet would you include in a preventive teaching plan for parents of young children?

   a.

   b.

   c.

   d.

e.

f.

D. Care for a child who is hospitalized as a result of maltreatment. Answer the following questions and include specific examples that illustrate these concepts.

1. Identify characteristics in each of the following areas that can be used to assess the vulnerability of families to abuse.

   a. Parents

   b. Child

   c. Environment

2. What two factors are used as diagnostic tools in determining child abuse?

   a.

   b.

3. Identify at least five areas that should arouse suspicion of abuse when the nurse is obtaining a history.

   a.

   b.

   c.

   d.

   e.

4. Develop three nursing diagnoses that could be used as a basis for the care of an abusing family.

   a.

   b.

   c.

5. Why are accurate nurse's notes essential to any suspected maltreatment situation?

6. For each of the following patient goals, identify one expected outcome that indicates achievement of these goals.

   a. Patient will experience no further abuse or neglect.

   b. Parents will exhibit evidence of positive interaction with children.

   c. Parents will exhibit knowledge of normal development.

7. Why should a nurse examine personal feelings related to the abuser and the victim in a domestic abuse situation?

Health Promotion of the School-Age Child and Family

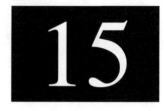

Chapter 15 discusses the school-age period, from age 6 through 12 years. Because this developmental stage is characterized by greater social awareness and social skills, it is important for nursing students to understand the roles of peer and family relationships, school, and play in the socialization process. At the completion of this chapter, the student will be able to use knowledge of the school-age child's growth and development to formulate nursing goals and interventions that foster health maintenance behavior in school-age children and their families.

REVIEW OF ESSENTIAL CONCEPTS

Promoting Optimum Growth and Development

1. What growth milestones mark the physiologic beginning and ending of the middle years (or school years)?

2. T F During the school-age years, a child will grow approximately 2 inches per year and will almost triple in weight.

3. Identify the three most pronounced physiologic changes that indicate increasing maturity in the school-age child.

   a.

   b.

   c.

4. The average age of puberty in girls is _____, and in boys it is _____ years.

5. According to Freud, the school-age child is in the _____ period.
   a. oral
   b. anal
   c. Oedipal
   d. latency

6. According to Erikson, the developmental task of middle childhood is acquiring a sense of:
   a. trust.
   b. autonomy.
   c. initiative.
   d. industry.

7. Failure to develop a sense of accomplishment results in a sense of _____.

8. T F Children with chronic physical or mental limitations may be at a disadvantage for acquisition of skills and are therefore at risk for feeling inferior.

9. According to Piaget, the school-age child is in the _____ stage.
   a. sensorimotor
   b. preoperational
   c. concrete operational
   d. formal operational

10. T   F   During this cognitive stage (answer to question 9), children progress from making judgments based on what they see (perceptual) to making judgments based on what they reason (conceptual).

11. One of the major cognitive tasks of school-age children is mastering the concept of

   _____.

12. Define the term *classification*.

13. T   F   The most significant skill acquired during the school-age years is the ability to read.

14. Which of the following best describes the younger (6- or 7-year-old) school-age child's perception of rules and judgment of actions?
   a. Judges an act by its intentions rather than by the consequences alone
   b. Believes that rules and judgments are not absolute
   c. Understands the reasons behind rules
   d. Interprets accidents and misfortunes as punishments for misdeeds

15. Which of the following best describes the older (10- to 12-year-old) school-age child's perception of rules and judgment of actions?
   a. Does not understand the reasons for rules
   b. Takes into account different points of view to make a judgment
   c. Judges an act by its consequences
   d. Believes that rules and judgments are absolute

16. The beliefs of _____ are more influential than those of _____ in matters of faith.

17. Identification with _____ _____ appears to be a very strong influence in the child's attainment of independence from parents.

18. Identify three valuable lessons that children learn from daily interactions with age-mates.

   a.

   b.

   c.

19. One of the outstanding characteristics of middle childhood is the formation of what groups?

20. _____ is the repetitive, persistent use of verbal behaviors by one or more _____ to inflict physical and/or psychological abuse.

21. Team play may contribute to what aspects of children's growth?

22. Define *self-concept*.

23. Until the child enters school, the primary sphere of influence is the _____.

24. _____ serve as role models with whom children identify and whom they try to emulate.

25. Children who spend some amount of time before or after school without supervision of an adult are termed

_____ _____.

26. During middle childhood, children may engage in antisocial behavior such as:

27. Identify the signs of stress school-age children may exhibit.

Promoting Optimum Health During the School Years

28. Match each behavior with the age at which it is typically exhibited.

    a. ____ Develops concept of numbers   1. 6 years

    b. ____ Enjoys group activities involving own sex but is beginning to mix with members of opposite sex   2. 9 years

                                                       3. 12 years

    c. ____ Enjoys group sports and organizations such as Girl Scouts/Boy Scouts

    d. ____ Loves friends; talks incessantly about them

29. What two factors are contributing to an increase in childhood obesity?

    a.

    b.

30. T F The appearance of permanent teeth in the school-age child begins with the eruption of the 6-year molar.

31. Before providing information on sexuality to parents and children, the nurse must first be knowledgeable about:

    a.

    b.

    c.

32. T F School nurses are vital to the development, implementation, and evaluation of health care plans for chronically ill or disabled children.

33. T F The most common cause of severe accidental injury and death in school-age children is motor vehicle accidents.

APPLYING CRITICAL THINKING TO NURSING PRACTICE

A. Jimmy Douglas, age 9 years, is brought to the pediatrician's office by his mother for his annual physical examination. His height and weight are obtained, and his height is 52 in (132.2 cm), and his weight is 62 lb (28.13 kg). His vision is evaluated as 20/30 in both eyes.

   1. Plot Jimmy's height and weight on a growth chart. How do his measurements compare with the norms for this age?

      a. Height

      b. Weight

   2. Mrs. Douglas tells the nurse that Jimmy likes to help his father with the yard work. However, Jimmy's work is not always up to his father's expectations. What advice could be given?

   3. Mrs. Douglas expresses concern because she is having a problem with dishonesty in her 6-year-old daughter. What information could the nurse provide to assist Mrs. Douglas in dealing with this concern?

B. Interview a school-age child and his parents about changing interpersonal relationships and peer groups. Answer the following questions and include specific responses to illustrate the concepts.

   1. Why do school-age children spend an increased amount of time away from their homes and families?

   2. Why are relationships with age-mates an important social interaction in the life of the school-age child?

   3. What would the nurse teach parents to prevent injury to the child from motor vehicle accidents?

     a.

     b.

     c.

     d.

     e.

   4. What would the nurse teach parents to prevent accidental drowning?

     a.

     b.

     c.

     d.

     e.

     f.

Health Promotion of the Adolescent and Family

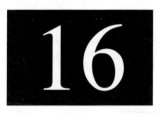

Chapter 16 examines the adolescent period, which is a difficult transition from childhood to adulthood. At the completion of this chapter, the student will understand the interplay of physical, psychosocial, and emotional factors in the adolescent's development and interpersonal relationships. This knowledge will enable the student to provide anticipatory guidance to assist the child and family with the intricate developmental issues of adolescence.

REVIEW OF ESSENTIAL CONCEPTS

Promoting Optimum Growth and Development

1. Adolescence begins with the gradual appearance of _____ _____ _____ and

   ends with cessation of _____ _____.

2. Differentiate between the following terms.

   a. Puberty

   b. Adolescence

3. The physical changes of puberty are primarily the result of _____ _____.

4. Identify the two most obvious physical changes that occur during adolescence.

   a.

   b.

5. Differentiate between the following two terms.

   a. Primary sex characteristics

   b. Secondary sex characteristics

6. _____ and _____ are the two types of sex hormones responsible for the variety of biologic changes observed during pubescence and puberty.

7. The normal age range for the onset of menarche is usually considered to be _____ to _____ years; the average age is _____ years.

8. The first pubescent changes in boys are _____ enlargement and the initial appearance of

   _____ _____.

9. Most of the physical growth of adolescents occurs during a 24- to 36-month period known as the adolescent

   _____ _____.

10. Skeletal growth differs between boys and girls. Match the following to reflect these differences accurately.

    a. ____ Greater overall height   1. Boys

    b. ____ Longer arms and legs   2. Girls

    c. ____ Greater shoulder width

    d. ____ Greater hip width

11. T   F   Enlargement of the larynx and vocal cords occurs in both boys and girls to produce voice changes.

12. _____ glands become extremely active during puberty, contributing to the pathogenesis of acne.

13. T   F   Adult values for the formed elements of the blood, respiratory rate, and basal metabolic rate are attained during adolescence.

14. According to Erikson, the developmental crisis of adolescence is developing a sense of:
    a. industry.
    b. identity.
    c. initiative.
    d. autonomy.

15. A sense of _____ identity appears to be an essential precursor to the sense of _____ identity.

16. When does role diffusion occur?

17. Adolescents encounter expectations for mature sex-role behavior from both _____ and

    _____.

18. Adolescents are unstable emotionally. They vacillate quickly between _____ behavior and

    _____ behavior.

19. According to Piaget, the adolescent is in the stage of _____ _____.

20. Identify five characteristics that are typical of the adolescent's thought processes.

    a.

    b.

    c.

    d.

    e.

21. The _____ _____ has more influence on an adolescent's self-evaluation and behavior than do parents.

22. Feelings of immortality, although viewed as negative, can serve as an important developmental function. This feeling can give adolescents courage to:

23. Statistics reveal that _____ of all teens have had sex by age 17.

24. Nurses need to recognize _____-_____ attraction and to be sensitive to the fact that not all youths are involved in heterosexual relationships.

25. T   F   It has been determined that the body image established during adolescence is temporary and subject to change.

26. All teenagers, regardless of gender, are very concerned with the question:

Promoting Optimum Health During Adolescence

27. The major causes of morbidity and mortality in adolescence are _____-_____

    _____.

28. T   F   The increase in height, weight, muscle mass, and sexual maturity of adolescence is accompanied by greater nutritional requirements.

29. Obesity is increasing in the adolescent in the United States. What are the two major contributing factors?

    a.

    b.

30. What type of visual disturbance is most common during adolescence?

31. List five major areas of stress for the adolescent.

    a.

    b.

    c.

    d.

    e.

32. T   F   Sex education instruction should be presented in a straightforward manner, using correct terminology.

33. The greatest single cause of death in the adolescent age group is _____ _____.

34. The single greatest cause of fatal injuries in adolescents is _____ _____

    _____.

35. The majority of fatal and nonfatal motor vehicle crashes involve the use of _____.

APPLYING CRITICAL THINKING TO NURSING PRACTICE

A. Alice Spears is a 14-year-old who comes to the pediatric clinic for a yearly checkup. She is accompanied by her mother. Although she has felt well recently, Alice is concerned because she is overweight and has recently developed acne. She also began menstruating 6 months ago.

    1. Alice's height is 64 in (162.7 cm), and her weight is 161 lb (73.08 kg). How do her measurements compare with those of other girls her age?

       a. Height

       b. Weight

2. What principles of physical growth should be explained to Alice since she is concerned about her weight?

B. Interview the parents of an adolescent about the teenager's involvement in peer groups, relationship with parents, and sense of identity. Answer the following questions and include specific responses that illustrate these concepts.

1. How does the peer group contribute to the development of a sense of identity in the adolescent?

2. Identify four ways in which group identity is demonstrated by the adolescent.

   a.

   b.

   c.

   d.

3. Why are peer groups an important influence during the adolescent years?

C. Interview an adolescent about his health promotion behavior. Answer the following questions, and include specific responses to illustrate these concepts.

1. Why is fatigue a common complaint of adolescence?

2. What can be gained from participation in sports?

   a.

   b.

   c.

3. Why should the nurse promote dental hygiene in the adolescent?

4. What developmental characteristics predispose the adolescent to accidents?

5. What are the most common types of accidents that occur during the adolescent years?

   a.

   b.

   c.

   d.

6. What elements should the nurse include in a sex education program for adolescents?

   a.

   b.

   c.

   d.

7. Because most adolescents tend to overeat or undereat, how can the nurse assist adolescents to select and stick to a nutritious diet?

   a.

   b.

   c.

   d.

Health Problems of School-Age Children and Adolescents

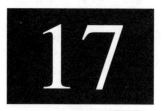

Chapter 17 introduces nursing considerations that are integral to the care of the school-age child and the adolescent experiencing physical health problems. Although this age group is usually healthy, students need to be aware of the common health problems related to the physical changes and other potentially serious illnesses or injuries that may affect this group. At the completion of this chapter, the student will understand the commonly encountered physical health deviations of the school-age child and the adolescent; recognize the potential for secondary psychologic problems; and be able to develop a nursing care plan to support the school-age child or adolescent and the family.

REVIEW OF ESSENTIAL CONCEPTS

Common Health Problems

1. The principal cause of infectious mononucleosis is the _____-_____ virus.

2. The early symptoms of mononucleosis are:

   a.

   b.

   c.

   d.

   e.

   f.

   g.

3. The _____, a slide test of high specificity, is used in the diagnosis of infectious mononucleosis.

4. Identify factors related to an adolescent's decision to begin smoking.

5. T   F   The use of smokeless tobacco products is a safe substitute for cigarette smoking.

6. Youth-to-Youth programs that emphasize the immediate _____ _____ _____ consequences of smoking are most effective in changing teenagers' attitudes toward smoking.

Health Problems Related to Sports Participation

7. Identify three examples of overuse syndromes.

   a.

   b.

   c.

8. Stress fractures occur as a result of:

9. The nurse's role in relation to sports injuries is directed toward:

   a.

   b.

   c.

   d.

10. T   F   Prevention of sports injuries is probably the most important aspect of any athletic program.

Altered Growth and Development

11. On a worldwide scale, the most common cause of short stature and/or developmental delay is

    _____ _____.

12. Girls with Turner syndrome may be diagnosed at puberty because they display three features:

    a.

    b.

    c.

13. The primary characteristic features of boys with Klinefelter syndrome include:

    a.

    b.

Disorders Related to the Reproductive System

14. T   F   The most common cause of secondary amenorrhea during adolescence is inhibition of the secretion of pituitary hormones.

15. The treatment of choice for dysmenorrhea in adolescents is the administration of nonsteroidal antiinflammatory drugs that block the formation of _____.

16. Young females need to be taught to wipe _____ to _____ after toileting to help prevent vaginitis.

17. The usual presenting symptom for testicular cancer is a heavy, hard, painless _____ on the

    _____.

18. All adolescent boys should be taught to perform _____ _____-

    _____ every month in order to detect testicular cancer early.

Health Problems Related to Sexuality

19. The most frequent complications of adolescent pregnancy are:

    a.

    b.

    c.

    d.

    e.

    f.

    g.

20. The choice of a safe and effective contraceptive method must be _____ _____ _____

    _____.

21. The most prevalent sexually transmitted diseases in the adolescent population are _____

    _____ _____ (_____) and _____.

22. The two sexually transmitted diseases that do not have a cure are:

    a.

    b.

23. Match the following sexually transmitted diseases with their causative organisms and the drug of choice for treatment. (Answers may be used more than once.)

a. ____   Gonorrhea

b. ____   Chlamydial infection

c. ____   Herpes pro genitalis

d. ____   Syphilis

e. ____   Trichomoniasis

1. *C. trachomatis*

2. Herpes simplex (HSV)

3. *Trichomonas vaginalis*

4. *Neisseria gonorrhoeae*

5. *Treponema pallidum*

6. Metronidazole

7. Doxycycline

8. Acyclovir

9. Penicillin

10. Ciproflaxin

24. Pelvic inflammatory disease in adolescents often results from untreated _____ or

_____ infections.

25. Name the complications of pelvic inflammatory disease that are of major concern.

26. During the initial contact with adolescent rape victims, it is important that they know they are:

a.

b.

27. The two phases of the rape trauma syndrome are:

a.

b.

28. The primary goal of nursing care for the rape victim is to:

Eating Disorders

29. A child is _____ when his or her BMI measurement exceeds the _____ percentile.

30. Obesity is caused by a variety of factors that include:

    a.

    b.

    c.

    d.

    e.

    f.

31. Theories that tend to explain the development of obesity are:

    a.

    b.

32. The goals of a weight-loss program include:

    a.

    b.

    c.

    d.

33. The key to success to lose weight is _____.

34. In the management of obesity, it has been observed that:
    a. weight loss will occur only when caloric expenditure is greater than caloric intake.
    b. there is little correlation between motivation to lose weight and the success of the weight-reduction program.
    c. the most successful diets are those that require the avoidance of specific foods.
    d. the alteration of eating behavior has little effect in maintaining long-term weight control.

35. T   F   The use of appetite-suppressant drugs is supported by practitioners as an effective therapy.

36. _____ _____ is a disorder characterized by a refusal to maintain a minimally normal body weight and severe weight loss in the absence of obvious physical causes.

37. The average age of onset of anorexia nervosa is _____ years of age.

38. The two dominant aspects of anorexia nervosa are:

    a.

    b.

39. List the clinical manifestations of anorexia nervosa.

    a.

    b.

    c.

    d.

    e.

    f.

    g.

    h.

40. Treatment of anorexia nervosa has three major thrusts:

    a.

    b.

    c.

41. _____ is an eating disorder characterized by binge eating.

42. Purging methods employed by bulimics include:

43. Briefly describe the two categories of bulimics.

    a.

    b.

44. T   F   Medical complications occur in bulimics primarily as a result of their frequent vomiting.

45. Identify two nursing interventions that are important during the acute phase of treatment of bulimia.

    a.

    b.

Disorders With Behavioral Components

46. Define *attention deficit hyperactivity disorder*.

47. List the components of the multiple approach to the management of attention deficit hyperactivity disorder.

    a.

    b.

    c.

    d.

    e.

48. Define *enuresis*.

49. List the various therapeutic techniques that can be employed to manage enuresis.

    a.

    b.

    c.

    d.

    e.

50. Define *encopresis*.

51. The characteristic symptoms of posttraumatic stress disorder are:

    a.

    b.

    c.

52. What are the three stages of response in posttraumatic stress disorder?

    a.

    b.

    c.

53. What is the primary nursing goal in the management of school phobia?

54. Recurrent abdominal pain is almost always attributed to a _____ etiology.

55. Define *conversion reaction*.

56. T   F   Depression in the child is easy to detect.

57. List behavioral characteristics of children with depression.

    a.

    b.

    c.

    d.

    e.

    f.

    g.

58. *Childhood schizophrenia* is a term used to describe severe deviation in _____ functioning.

Serious Health Problems of Later Childhood and Adolescence

59. T   F   Most drug use begins with experimentation.

60. Complete the following statements related to substance abuse.

    a. _____ is a socially accepted depressant that most noticeably affects the

       _____ _____ system.

    b. _____ is a purer and more menacing form of cocaine.

c. Addiction to narcotic drugs brings an additional risk for _____ and _____ infection because of self-neglect and contamination of needles.

d. _____ produces an excitement more intense than cocaine.

e. _____ of glue and other volatile substances is dangerous because respiratory arrest can occur easily.

61. A major factor in the treatment and rehabilitation of the young drug user is careful assessment to determine the _____ the drug plays in the youngster's life.

62. T   F   Suicide is the third leading cause of death during the adolescent years.

63. Distinguish between the following terms.

a. Suicide ideation

b. Parasuicide

64. The method of choice for most adolescents who attempt suicide is _____

_____.

65. T   F   Most adolescents' suicidal threats are not to be taken seriously.

66. Nursing care of the suicidal adolescent includes:

a.

b.

c.

67. The most important aspect of management is the _____ of warning signs that a youngster is troubled and may attempt suicide.

APPLYING CRITICAL THINKING TO NURSING PRACTICE

A. Rosemary, age 16 years, is admitted to the adolescent unit with a severe sore throat, persistent fever, fatigue, and general malaise. A diagnosis of infectious mononucleosis is made.

1. How was the diagnosis of infectious mononucleosis established?

2. What might the nurse tell Rosemary about the usual course of infectious mononucleosis in the following areas?

   a. Acute symptoms disappear:

   b. Persistent fatigue subsides:

   c. Restrict activity for:

3. What therapeutic measures may be used to relieve Rosemary's sore throat?

4. What are the nursing goals in caring for Rosemary?

   a.

   b.

B. Derek, age 15 years, has been experiencing a deep, persistent, dull ache over the left tibia that progressed to pain with each heel strike during a cross-country meet. The coach refers Derek to the sports medicine team at University Medical Center for evaluation. A stress fracture of the left tibia is discovered.

1. What is the major goal of the therapeutic management of overuse syndromes such as Derek's stress fracture?

2. Derek asks the nurse on the sports medicine team whether she thinks running is a good sport for him to continue in the future. What should the nurse assess to answer this question?

3. What nursing interventions might the nurse together with the coaches and athletic trainers employ?

   a.

   b.

   c.

   d.

C. Spend a day in a gynecology clinic to oversee the diseases and disorders affecting the female reproductive system. Answer the following questions and include specific examples to illustrate these concepts.

1. In secondary amenorrhea, if pregnancy was ruled out as the cause, what other data would you evaluate from the history of the patient as the most probable etiologies?

2. The first-line treatment for adolescents with dysmenorrhea is:

3. The nursing responsibilities in relation to sexually transmitted disease are all-encompassing. For each of the following nursing goals, identify one appropriate intervention to accomplish this goal.

a. Education of patient

b. Primary prevention of STDs

c. Tertiary prevention through treatment

D. Interview an obese adolescent to assess eating patterns. Answer the following questions and include specific responses that illustrate these concepts.

1. Why is obesity considered a major problem of adolescence?

2. Formulate five nursing diagnoses that could apply to the obese adolescent.

a.

b.

c.

d.

e.

3. What nursing goals should be included in a weight-loss program?

a.

b.

c.

d.

E.   Role-play an interaction between a nurse and an anorexic or bulimic adolescent to demonstrate the adolescent's perception of the disorder and how the nurse would provide counseling.

1. What usually precedes the onset of anorexia nervosa?

2. What contemporary trends are considered factors in the greatly increased incidence of anorexia and bulimia?

a.

b.

3. The following are characteristics associated with anorexia nervosa and/or bulimia. Mark "A" if the item is related to anorexia, "B" if it applies to bulimia, and "A, B" if it may be associated with both disorders.

a. ____   Binge eating

b. ____   Self-induced vomiting

c. ____   Self-imposed starvation

d. ____   Cold intolerance

e. ____   Sometimes normal or slightly above normal weight

f. ____   Emaciated appearance

g. ____   Increased incidence of dental caries

F.   Michelle is a 16-year-old girl admitted to the adolescent unit following the ingestion of ten of her mother's barbiturates with an unknown quantity of alcohol. Michelle is known to be a "problem drinker." When she recovers consciousness after gastric lavage, Michelle sobs that she wishes she were dead because she has broken up with her boyfriend.

1. In what ways was Michelle's suicide attempt a typical one for an adolescent girl?

2. In assessing Michelle's family status, what factors might the nurse likely discover?

3. The most important nursing interventions for Michelle and her family to prevent further suicide attempts would include:

Chronic Illness, Disability, or End-of-Life Care for the Child and Family

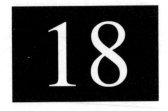

Chapter 18 introduces nursing considerations essential to the care of the child with a chronic illness or a disability or the child who is terminally ill. At the completion of this chapter, the student will understand the impact that a diagnosis of a chronic illness or disability has on both the child and family and be able to develop appropriate nursing interventions to assist each family member to adjust and develop to his or her fullest potential despite the disability. The student will also be able to provide care at the end of life that meets the physical, psychologic, emotional, and spiritual needs of the child and family.

REVIEW OF ESSENTIAL CONCEPTS

Perspectives in the Care of Children With Special Needs

1. Define *children with special needs*.

2. Match each term with its definition.

   a. ___ Chronic illness

   b. ___ Disability

   c. ___ Developmental disability

   d. ___ Handicap

   1. Functional limitation that interferes with a person's ability to walk, lift, hear, or learn

   2. A condition or barrier imposed by society, the environment, or one's self; not a synonym for disability

   3. A condition that interferes with daily functioning for more than 3 months in a year, causes hospitalization of more than 1 month in a year, or is likely to do either of these

   4. Any mental and/or physical disability that is manifested before the age of 22 years and is likely to continue indefinitely

3. Identify and explain the changing trends in the care of children with special needs.

   a. Developmental focus

   b. Family-centered care

119

4. Consistent with normalization, children with special needs are discharged earlier to the home environment. Home care is guided by three goals. List them.

   a.

   b.

   c.

5. _____ refers to the integration of children with special needs into regular classrooms.

The Family of the Child With Special Needs

6. List the adaptive tasks of parents who have children with chronic conditions.

   a.

   b.

   c.

   d.

   e.

   f.

   g.

   h.

7. T   F   Fathers and mothers of children with special needs adjust and cope differently.

8. List at least three ways parents can promote healthy sibling relationships with children with special needs.

   a.

   b.

   c.

9. _____ is a process of recognizing, promoting, and enhancing competence.

10. List the sequence of stages through which a family progresses following the diagnosis of a chronic illness or disability.

   a.

   b.

   c.

11. The four most common responses manifested during the adjustment stage are:

    a.

    b.

    c.

    d.

12. Describe the four types of parental reactions to the child that may occur during the period of adjustment.

    a. Overprotection

    b. Rejection

    c. Denial

    d. Gradual acceptance

13. Explain the concept of chronic sorrow.

14. Explain the concept of family adjustment referred to as *functional burden*.

The Child With Special Needs

15. Identify five variables that influence a child's reaction to chronic illness or disability.

    a.

    b.

c.

d.

e.

16. T   F   The impact of a chronic illness or disability is influenced by the age of onset.

17. Identify the coping patterns used by the child with special needs.

a.

b.

c.

d.

e.

Nursing Care of the Family and Child With Special Needs

18. List the factors the nurse would assess to determine the family's adjustment to the birth of a child with special needs.

a.

b.

c.

d.

e.

19. List the three most common responses of families to the diagnosis of a disability.

a.

b.

c.

20. In order to construct a nursing plan of care for the child with special needs, the nurse must observe the following regarding the child:

a.

b.

c.

21. One of the most important interventions is alleviating the child's feelings of being different and normalizing his or her life. What guidelines would promote normalization?

    a.

    b.

    c.

    d.

    e.

22. One of the most important aspects of promoting normal development is to encourage the child's:

23. To foster a realistic adjustment of the family with a special-needs child, the nurse must educate the family. This education should include the importance of discipline. What purposes are served by discipline?

24. One of the most difficult adjustments of parents with a special-needs child is the ability to set

    _____ _____ _____ for the child.

Perspectives on the Care of Children at the End of Life

25. The World Health Organization, in its definition of *palliative care*, states the goal of palliative care to be:

26. T   F   The ANA Code for Nurses supports the active intent on the part of a nurse to end a person's life (euthanasia).

27. For the preschool child, the greatest fear concerning death is:

28. Describe the goal of hospice care for children.

Nursing Care of the Child and Family at the End of Life

29. The terminally ill child and family usually experience the following fears:

    a.

    b.

    c.

30. Siblings of the dying child may become resentful of their sick sibling and begin to feel _____ or

    _____ about their feelings.

31. Identify the major areas that are symptoms of normal grief.

    a.

    b.

    c.

    d.

    e.

32. It is important for families to know that mourning may _____ _____.

33. Identify the strategies the nurse can use to maintain the ability to work effectively with terminally ill children.

    a.

    b.

    c.

    d.

    e.

    f.

    g.

APPLYING CRITICAL THINKING TO NURSING PRACTICE

A. Spend a morning at a clinic or school for children with disabilities to observe various treatment modalities and programs. Answer the following questions and include specific examples to illustrate these concepts.

    1. Describe the four major changes that have occurred in the provision of services to children with special needs.

        a.

        b.

        c.

        d.

    2. How have the changes above served to improve the care of children with special needs?

        a.

        b.

        c.

        d.

B. Care for a child who has recently been diagnosed as having a chronic illness or disability.

    1. Briefly describe the stages through which a family progresses following the diagnosis of a chronic illness or disability.

        a. Shock and denial

        b. Adjustment

        c. Reintegration and acknowledgment

    2. List nine examples of behavior that should alert the nurse to the presence of denial.

        a.

        b.

c.

d.

e.

f.

g.

h.

i.

3. Why is it important for the nurse to allow denial to occur for a reasonable period?

a. In parents

b. In the child

4. The nurse observes the 5-year-old sister of a child with cystic fibrosis behaving as follows: withdrawn, irritable, throwing toys across the room. What would you tell the concerned mother to do?

C. Interview the parents of a child with a disability to determine the family's adjustment. Answer the following questions and include specific responses to illustrate these concepts.

1. Identify the areas the nurse should assess when determining the adequacy of a family's support systems.

a.

b.

c.

2. Why is it necessary for the nurse to assess the family's specific perceptions concerning the illness or disability?

3. Briefly describe some of the behaviors that might be observed in a child who has coped with a disability.

   a.

   b.

   c.

4. What are the basic nursing goals for families and children with special needs?

   a.

   b.

   c.

   d.

   e.

   f.

5. List outcomes the nurse would expect to observe if the following patient (family) goal is achieved: "Will exhibit positive adjustment behaviors to the diagnosis."

D. Interview children in various age groups to determine their perceptions of death. Answer the following questions, and include specific responses to illustrate these concepts.

   1. How do children between the ages of 3 and 5 years view death?

      a.

      b.

      c.

      d.

2. If a preschooler becomes seriously ill, how is he or she likely to perceive the illness?

3. By _____ or _____ years of age, most children have an adult concept of death.

4. Identify at least five nursing interventions that could be used when caring for a terminally ill adolescent in the hospital.

a.

b.

c.

d.

e.

E. Care for a child who has a terminal illness and the child's family.

1. List nursing goals that would address the nursing diagnosis "Altered growth and development related to terminal illness and/or impending death."

a.

b.

c.

2. List evaluation data that would reflect the meeting of the goal "Support child during terminal phase."

a.

b.

3. The nurse could implement which of the following interventions after observing that the parents of a terminally ill child were not visiting very frequently?
a. Warn the parents that if they do not visit their child frequently now, they may experience intense guilt feelings after death.
b. Tell the child it is good to have time alone to think about death and to prepare for this new experience.
c. Call the parents in and ask them to explain why they are not visiting frequently.
d. Spend as much time with the child as possible, recognizing that the parents may need to withdraw temporarily to cope.

Impact of Cognitive or Sensory Impairment on the Child and Family

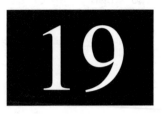

Chapter 19 introduces nursing considerations essential to the care of the child with a cognitive impairment or a sensory or communication disorder. Since these deficits pose a special threat to the child's developmental potential, it is important for students to understand the nuances of care of children with these types of disorders. This knowledge will enable the student to develop nursing strategies that will promote optimum achievement of the child's potential.

REVIEW OF ESSENTIAL CONCEPTS

Cognitive Impairment

1. Define *mental retardation*.

2. When is a diagnosis of cognitive impairment usually made?

3. Four dimensions of care for mental retardation are considered in the classification of the mentally retarded in addition to IQ; they are:

   a.

   b.

   c.

   d.

4. What does EMR stand for?

5. List the four classifications of mental retardation.

   a.

   b.

   c.

   d.

6. Identify the three causes of severe mental retardation.

   a.

   b.

   c.

7. _____ _____ _____ are valuable educational experiences for cognitively impaired children.

8. Describe the Education of the Handicapped Act (PL 101-476).

9. What two principles should guide the nurse when teaching self-help skills?

   a.

   b.

10. Toys are selected according to their _____ and _____ value.

11. _____ is a major consideration in selecting recreational and exercise activities.

12. Discipline must begin early. Limit-setting needs to be _____, applied _____, and be _____ for the child's mental age.

13. Parents must be assisted in teaching their mentally retarded adolescent how to deal with emerging sexuality. Because of the adolescent's easy persuasion and lack of judgment, what is the guiding principle you would tell the parents to use in their teaching?

14. Approximately 95% of all cases of Down syndrome are attributable to an extra chromosome _____.

15. How is the presence of Down syndrome confirmed?

16. What factor contributes to the development of respiratory difficulties in children with Down syndrome?

17. A significant percentage of Down syndrome children also have _____ defects.

18. The second most common genetic cause of mental retardation is _____ syndrome.

Sensory Impairment

19. Differentiate among the following terms.

   a. Hearing impaired

   b. Deaf

   c. Hard-of-hearing

20. List the causes of hearing impairment.

   a.

   b.

   c.

   d.

   e.

   f.

   g.

   h.

   i.

21. Differentiate among the following terms used to describe receptive-expressive disorders due to an organic central auditory defect.

   a. Aphasia

   b. Agnosia

c. Dysacusis

22. Hearing impairment is expressed in terms of _____, a unit of loudness.

23. One of the most common problems with hearing aids is _____ _____, an annoying whistling sound usually caused by improper fit of the ear mold.

24. Conductive hearing loss can be improved with the use of a _____ _____ to amplify sound.

25. _____ _____ can help profoundly deaf children to hear. It is important to use these

    devices at the _____ age possible, usually by _____ months of age.

26. When is an individual considered to be legally blind?

27. _____ _____ are the most common causes of visual impairment in children.

28. T   F   Refractive errors are evaluated by testing visual acuity.

29. Match each type of refractive error with its defining characteristics. (Answers may be used more than once.)

    a. ____ Myopia   1. Also referred to as *farsightedness*

    b. ____ Hyperopia   2. Also referred to as *nearsightedness*

    c. ____ Anisometropia   3. Refers to unequal curvatures in the cornea or lens so that light rays
                                          are bent in different directions, producing a blurred image
    d. ____ Astigmatism
                                       4. Refers to the ability to see objects clearly at close range but not at a
                                          distance

                                       5. Refers to a difference of refractive strength in each eye

                                       6. Specially ground lenses used in correction of defect

                                       7. Refers to the ability to see objects clearly at a distance

                                       8. Biconcave lenses used in correction of defect

                                       9. Treated with corrective lenses to improve vision in each eye so that
                                          the eyes work as a unit

                                       10. Convex lenses used in correction of defect

                                       11. Often results in child squinting in an attempt to try to correct the
                                           defect

30. Define *amblyopia*.

31. _____ refers to malalignment of the eyes.

32. What occurs when there is a malalignment of the eyes?

33. The definition "inward deviation of the eye" refers to a type of strabismus that is properly termed

    _____.

34. Define the following terms.

    a. Cataract

    b. Glaucoma

35. Why are mobility and locomotion skills typically delayed in blind children?

36. What is the most traumatic sensory impairment?

37. Describe the effects that auditory and visual impairment have on the child's development.

38. _____ is a congenital malignant tumor arising from the retina.

39. The symptom of retinoblastoma that is first observed as "a whitish glow in the pupil" is known as the

    _____ _____ _____.

40. The overall prognosis for retinoblastoma is approximately a _____ survival rate.

41. A hallmark characteristic of autism is:
    a. increased quality of social interaction.
    b. inability to maintain eye contact.
    c. advanced language development.
    d. no unusual motor mannerisms noted.

APPLYING CRITICAL THINKING TO NURSING PRACTICE

A. Spend a day in an early intervention unit to observe the various methods used in the management of the child with cognitive impairment.

1. The major intervention for the prevention of mental retardation is _____

   _____ _____ for the small premature infant and other high-risk newborns.

2. What are the major nursing goals of caring for children with mental retardation in relation to the nursing diagnosis "Altered growth and development related to impaired cognitive functioning"?

   a.

   b.

3. What areas should the nurse assess when a child with cognitive impairment is hospitalized?

   a.

   b.

   c.

   d.

   e.

   f.

4. Identify two nursing diagnoses appropriate for caring for a child with mental retardation.

   a.

   b.

5. What is the rationale for the intervention "Help family set realistic goals for child"?

6. List the expected outcomes for the goal "Will be prepared for long-term care of the child."

   a.

   b.

B. Interview the parents of a child with Down syndrome to identify the major management problems related to this disorder. Answer the following questions and include specific responses to illustrate these concepts.

1. What is the nurse's role when parents are informed of a diagnosis of Down syndrome in their child?

   a.

   b.

   c.

   d.

2. List the physical characteristics that may cause management problems for these parents, thus requiring education.

   a.

   b.

   c.

   d.

   e.

   f.

C. Spend a day in a hearing clinic to observe testing, evaluation, and treatment modalities for the child with a hearing impairment. Answer the following questions and include specific examples to illustrate these concepts.

1. For each of the following nursing goals, list at least three nursing interventions that would be used when caring for a child with a hearing impairment and the family.

   a. Prevention of hearing loss

   b. Detection of hearing loss

2. What areas should the nurse assess when evaluating a child for a possible hearing loss?

   a. Infancy

    b. Childhood

  3. List the nursing goals that will address the nursing diagnosis "Altered growth and development related to impaired communication."

    a.

    b.

    c.

D. Spend a morning in a vision clinic to observe testing, evaluation, and treatment modalities for the child with a visual impairment. Answer the following questions and include specific examples to illustrate these concepts.

  1. A critical nursing responsibility is to assess children for possible visual impairment. Appropriate assessment involves:

    a.

    b.

    c.

  2. Identify four nursing goals for care of the child with visual impairment and the child's family.

    a.

    b.

    c.

    d.

  3. When the nurse is counseling the parents of an infant who is blind, what interventions would accomplish the goal "Promote parent-child attachment"?

    a.

    b.

E. Harry, age 17 months, is admitted for treatment of a retinoblastoma.

  1. If Harry is to have an enucleation of his affected eye, how would the nurse prepare his parents for the child's postoperative appearance?

2. Because this defect is inherited, the nurse would encourage Harry's parents to:

F.   Care for a child with autism.

1. The child's intellectual functioning is assessed. The majority of autistic children are:

2. List the nursing goals used in the management of autism.

a.

b.

c.

d.

Family-Centered Home Care

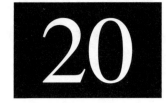

Chapter 20 presents important concepts related to family-centered home care, discharge planning, case management, and promotion of optimum development in the home care setting. At the completion of this chapter, the student will have knowledge of the components of effective home care and the importance of parent-professional and family-to-family collaboration. This knowledge will enable the student to use the nursing process to develop plans for safe, appropriate, and effective home care delivery.

REVIEW OF ESSENTIAL CONCEPTS

General Concepts of Home Care

1. The driving force in the efforts to move technology-dependent children from the hospital to the home setting

   is improving the quality of _____ for both the child and the _____.

2. The _____ of home care is less than that of hospital care for children dependent on medical technology and children requiring complex care.

3. With increased demand for nurses in home health and continued short supply of nurses, there has been an

   increased focus on the role of _____ _____.

4. What factors are contributing to the shortage of nurses for children in the home care setting?

   a.

   b.

   c.

5. Discharge planning for home care must begin early, be a _____ process, and involve

   the _____.

6. T   F   One family member should learn and demonstrate all aspects of the child's care in the hospital as part of discharge planning.

7. An in-hospital _____ period during which parents provide total care is beneficial; this may be

   followed by taking the child home on a brief _____ before final discharge planning.

8. List the five advantages of a predischarge home visit by the home care nurse.

   a.

   b.

c.

d.

e.

9. Optimum home care of the technologically dependent child requires case management to be viewed more

broadly as _____ _____.

10. What is the primary goal of coordination of care?

11. What three purposes should be served by coordinating care among multiple providers?

a.

b.

c.

12. Care coordination should promote the _____ role as primary decision maker and enhance the

_____ capability to meet the special needs of the child and the family unit.

13. The home care nurse must share a level of _____ expertise with a critical care nurse while

also being able to _____ equipment, procedures, and the nursing process to the home setting.

14. What five additional qualities are needed by the pediatric home care nurse?

a.

b.

c.

d.

e.

15. Nurses in pediatric home health face _____ (increasing, decreasing) demands for providing

high-quality care with _____ (more, fewer) resources in order to achieve positive patient outcomes.

Family-Centered Home Care

16. Regardless of the family's background, family _____ must be respected in the provision of
home care services.

17. State the key component of family-centered care that provides the philosophic basis for family-centered home care practice.

18. T   F   Believing that no one knows the child better than the family does is critical to the success of any home care plan.

19. What five broad areas of diversity need to be respected in providing home care?

    a.

    b.

    c.

    d.

    e.

20. The culturally sensitive nurse has the central goal of nursing care of the child and family of

    _____ _____.

21. Family-centered nursing practice is built on a foundation of parent-professional

    _____.

22. Communication with the family should not be _____, and families must be assured that they

    have a right to expect _____ in regard to the data collected about them.

23. Nurses should respect _____ preferences in any situation that will not pose danger or risk for the child.

Nursing Process

24. In the home, the _____ is a partner in each step of the nursing process, and all the information gathered as part of the assessment process is shared with the _____.

25. Family _____ should guide the planning process.

26. Both short-term and long-term goals should be outlined and agreed upon by the _____,

    _____, and _____ involved.

Promotion of Optimum Development, Self-Care, and Education

27. Throughout the developmental stages, a child's medical condition and dependence on medical technology

    may constrain and challenge normal _____.

28. List the four ways in which home care plans are designed to promote optimum development.

    a.

    b.

    c.

    d.

29. The extent to which a child is involved in his or her own care depends on what four factors?

    a.

    b.

    c.

    d.

30. The frame of reference for self-care in activities of daily living should be the goal of attaining _____-

    _____ competence.

31 Each family is entitled to an _____ _____ _____ _____
    (IFSP) to help ensure early intervention.

32. The _____ and _____ companies must be notified that this family is on a priority
    list when services are interrupted.

33. Before hospital discharge, _____ protocols should be developed and reviewed with both

    the _____ and professional caregivers.

34. T   F   The activity level and curiosity of young children do not raise additional safety considerations in
             the home care of technologically dependent children.

35. What time of day poses particular safety problems in the home care setting?

Family-to-Family Support

36. Family-to-family support is a unique source promoting family _____ through shared

    _____.

37. School-age children and adolescents just want to be _____ by their peers.

APPLYING CRITICAL THINKING TO NURSING PRACTICE

A. Jonathan, an 8-year-old with cerebral palsy, will be discharged to home care in 1 week. Prior to this admission, Jonathan had been receiving limited home care visits for range-of-motion exercises and gastrostomy tube feedings. During this admission, he has had a tracheostomy. He will require suctioning and oxygen p.r.n. His parents are anxious about their ability to care for Jonathan at home because of these additional care requirements.

1. What are some of the areas that the nurse responsible for discharge planning must address?

   a.

   b.

   c.

   d.

   e.

   f.

2. What are two possible approaches that could help Jonathan's parents develop new caregiving skills and confidence in their abilities?

   a.

   b.

3. In addition to providing direct care for Jonathan, what are the two areas of teaching responsibility of the home health care nurse during the first few days after discharge?

   a.

   b.

4. The home care agency case manager coordinates Jonathan's ongoing care. What needs and issues of the child and family must be addressed through care coordination?

   a. Needs of the child

   b. Issues of the child and family

B. Spend a day in the home of a family receiving home care for a child with complex medical needs. Observe the home care nurse's caregiving activities and the interactions between the nurse and the family. Answer the following questions and provide specific examples that illustrate these concepts.

1. How can much of the information needed to care for the child be collected?

2. What is the home care nurse's responsibility when communications among family members are overheard?

3. When disagreement arises between the parents and the home care nurse regarding proper procedures for the child's care, what should the nurse do in each of the following situations?

   a. A situation that will not pose danger or risk for the child

   b. A disagreement that cannot be resolved

   c. Parental desire to alter a treatment plan that is part of medical orders

4. The ultimate responsibility for managing the child's health, developmental, and emotional needs lies with the family. The three central concepts of this model are:

   a.

   b.

   c.

C. As a student, spend a day with a home care nurse who is caring for a 5-year-old boy who is technologically dependent. Observe the child, the setting, the family, and the nurse. Answer the following questions and give examples where necessary.

1. What interventions did you observe that would enhance normal development of self-esteem in this child?

   a.

   b.

   c.

2. This child has a sister who is a toddler. What safety considerations should have been in place to protect the toddler?

   a.

   b.

   c.

   d.

   e.

Family-Centered Care of the Child During Illness and Hospitalization

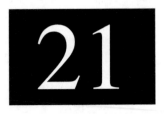

Chapter 21 provides an overview of how children of various ages react to illness, pain, and hospitalization. Children are extremely vulnerable to the stress of such experiences and respond to these stressors in a manner consistent with their developmental level. At the completion of this chapter, the student will be aware of how the child and family react to the stress of illness, pain, and hospitalization and will be able to intervene to lessen the trauma of these experiences.

REVIEW OF ESSENTIAL CONCEPTS

Stressors of Hospitalization and Children's Reactions

1. Children are vulnerable to the stress of illness and hospitalization because:

   a.

   b.

2. What five factors affect the child's reaction to the stress of hospitalization?

   a.

   b.

   c.

   d.

   e.

3. From middle infancy through preschool years, _____ is the major stressor related to hospitalization.

4. The three phases in the crisis of separation are _____, _____, and

   _____.

5. Adolescents experience the stress of separation primarily from their _____ rather than from their family.

6. The three major areas in which children experience loss of control are:

   a.

   b.

   c.

7. The needs of children vary with age. Match each of the following responses to loss of control with the age group the response exemplifies.

   a. ____ They strive for autonomy and react with negativism to any physical restriction.

   b. ____ The same feelings that make them feel omnipotent also make them feel out of control.

   c. ____ Explanations are understood only in terms of real events.

   d. ____ Their initial reaction to dependency is negativism and aggression.

   e. ____ They respond with depression, hostility, and frustration to physical restrictions.

   f. ____ They often voluntarily isolate themselves from age-mates until they can compete on an equal basis.

   g. ____ Altering of routine and ritual results in regression.

   h. ____ Any threat to their sense of identity results in a loss of control.

   i. ____ They are particularly vulnerable to feelings of loss of control because they are striving for independence and productivity.

   j. ____ They perceive illness or hospitalization as punishment for real or imagined misdeeds.

1. Toddlers

2. Preschoolers

3. School-age children

4. Adolescents

8. Identify each of the following statements regarding bodily injury and pain in children as true or false.

   a. T F A young infant's general reaction to painful stimuli is body movement associated with brief, loud crying.

   b. T F Toddlers are able to describe the type or intensity of the pain.

   c. T F Preschoolers' primary reaction to the stress of pain and fear is aggression.

   d. T F Distraction is an effective intervention for pain in infants.

   e. T F School-age children use passive methods of dealing with pain.

   f. T F Behaviors indicating pain in the toddler are grimacing, clenching teeth or lips, opening eyes wide, rocking, rubbing, and aggressiveness.

   g. T F Adolescents react to pain with resistance and aggression.

9. List the individual risk factors that increase the child's vulnerability to the stresses of hospitalization.

   a.

   b.

   c.

d.

e.

f.

Stressors and Reactions of the Family of the Child Who Is Hospitalized

10. Parents respond to the illness and hospitalization of their child in a fairly consistent manner. What are the stages of reaction?

a.

b.

c.

d.

11. The siblings of the hospitalized child may react with feelings of:

Nursing Care of the Child Who Is Hospitalized

12. Programs to prepare the child and family for the hospitalization experience are based on what principle?

13. The patient admission assessment should be individualized and should include an evaluation of:

a.

b.

c.

d.

e.

14. Once the assessment and history are collected, the information (data) must be applied to the

_____ _____ and communicated to other staff.

15. A primary nursing goal when a child is hospitalized (particularly children 5 years old or younger) is to

prevent effects of _____.

16. In order to prevent separation effects from hospitalization, many children's hospitals have shifted their policy to a _____-_____ care model.

17. Feelings of loss of control result from:

    a.

    b.

    c.

    d.

    e.

18. The four actions that the nurse can take to minimize feelings of loss of control are:

    a.

    b.

    c.

    d.

19. T   F   Infants and children are adequately medicated for pain.

20. The (AHCPR) _____ _____ _____ _____ _____ _____

    _____ has published clinical guidelines developed by pain experts that focus on the management of all types of pain.

21. An operational definition of *pain* that is useful in clinical practice is:

22. Identify the fallacies or myths regarding pain relief in children.

    a.

    b.

    c.

d.

e.

f.

g.

23. Define the following terms that are used in relation to opioid addiction:

    a. Physical dependence

    b. Tolerance

    c. Addiction

24. QUESTT is an approach to pain assessment in children. Identify the components of this approach.

    a. Q =

    b. U =

    c. E =

    d. S =

    e. T =

    f. T =

25. The seven scales that are appropriate to use in assessing pain in children are:

    a.

    b.

    c.

    d.

    e.

    f.

    g.

26. Identify the seven scales that use behavioral and physiological parameters to measure pain in young non-verbal children.

    a.

    b.

    c.

    d.

    e.

    f.

    g.

27. List the nonpharmacologic strategies suggested to relieve pain.

28. When using pharmacologic methods to control pain, what are the four "rights" that must be considered?

    a.

    b.

    c.

    d.

29. _____ (_____) is not recommended as a first-line opioid analgesic for the management of any kind of pain in children.

30. When opioids are combined with other drugs for pain relief, these other drugs are termed

    _____.

31. A common drug combination is known as DPT. What drugs are included?

32. Drugs that are used in combination with opioids to control pain symptoms (they may or may not have anal-

    gesic properties) are termed _____ _____ or

    _____ .

33. Define the term *equianalgesia*.

34. A significant advance in the administration of intravenous analgesics is the use of _____-

    _____ _____ (_____).

35. Another new route for drug administration that is enhancing pain management is _____ analge-
    sia.

36. EMLA is _____ _____ of _____ _____ .

37. For the most effective control of continuous pain, the _____-_____-_____

    (_____) method is used.

38. The most serious side effect of opioids is _____ _____ .

39. The most common side effect of opioids is _____ .

40. Play is the _____ of children.

41. Match each type of play with its description or purpose.

    a. ____   Offers the best opportunity for emotional   1. Play therapy
              expression, including the release of anger
                                                                  2. Therapeutic play
    b. ____   A psychologic technique reserved for use by
              trained therapists as an interpretative method   3. Dramatic play

    c. ____   Nondirective method for helping children deal   4. Expressive activities
              with their concerns and fears

    d. ____   Allows children to reenact frightening or
              puzzling hospital experiences

Nursing Care of the Family

42. List the main goals for nursing care of the family.

    a.

    b.

    c.

    d.

Care of the Child and Family in Special Hospital Situations

43. The advantages of ambulatory care are:

    a.

    b.

    c.

44. Stressors for the child and family when in the neonatal or pediatric ICU can be grouped into what four categories?

    a.

    b.

    c.

    d.

APPLYING CRITICAL THINKING TO NURSING PRACTICE

A. Ronik, age 2 years, is admitted to the pediatric unit with a diagnosis of meningitis. When his parents briefly leave the room, Ronik begins to shake the bars of the crib, to scream and cry loudly, and to refuse attention from the nurse.

    1. When the nurse assesses Ronik's behavior, she knows it is characteristic of the _____ stage of separation.

    2. List at least one appropriate intervention to deal with Ronik's behavior.

B. Amy, 2 years old, is admitted to the pediatric unit for evaluation and treatment of a urinary tract infection. Both Amy and her parents appear anxious.

    1. In order to maintain contact between Amy and her parents and siblings, identify at least one appropriate nursing intervention.

2. Identify at least two nursing interventions to accomplish the nursing goal of minimizing the effects of loss of control.

   a.

   b.

C. Robert, age 4 years, is admitted to the pediatric unit with a diagnosis of gastroenteritis.

   1. List the primary nursing goals for support of the family of a hospitalized child.

      a.

      b.

      c.

      d.

   2. List at least three nursing interventions to accomplish the nursing goal "Will receive adequate support."

      a.

      b.

      c.

   3. List at least three nursing interventions to accomplish the nursing goal "Will experience positive relationships."

      a.

      b.

      c.

   4. Robert's mother asks you, the nurse, for advice on what toys she should bring to her child. With consideration for developmental needs and for safety, what types of toys would you recommend?

   5. What outcomes would reflect the attainment of the nursing goal "Will demonstrate knowledge of home care"?

      a.

      b.

D. Manuel, age 6 years, is being admitted to the pediatric unit with a complaint of abdominal pain.

   1. What steps (interventions) should the nurse follow when admitting Manuel to the unit?

      a.

      b.

      c.

   2. In order to assess Manuel's pain, what pain assessment scales would be suitable?

      a.

      b.

      c.

      d.

      e.

      f.

   3. Manuel's morphine order reads: Morphine 0.20 mg IV q 3–4 hours p.r.n. How would you administer this medication for maximum effect?

   4. What two side effects of morphine would you assess for?

      a.

      b.

Pediatric Variations of Nursing Intervention

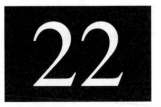

Chapter 22 provides an overview of the modifications to nursing procedures that must be implemented when working with children. Since children differ from adults in biologic, cognitive, and emotional function and response, nursing practice must be altered to meet the special needs of the pediatric patient. Small children who are hospitalized are separated from their usual environment and do not possess the capacity for abstract thinking and reasoning, which has ramifications both for compliance and for safety. At the completion of this chapter, the student will have the theoretical basis to be able to safely implement nursing procedures with the pediatric population.

REVIEW OF ESSENTIAL CONCEPTS

General Concepts Related to Pediatric Procedures

1. What is informed consent?

2. Three conditions must be met for an informed consent to be valid. What are they?

   a.

   b.

   c.

3. In relation to informed consent, the nurse should know the state law regarding an emancipated or mature minor, as well as the age of majority. Define the following:

   a. Mature minor

   b. Emancipated minor

4. Children, regardless of their ages, require psychologic _____ to minimize the fear and discomfort experienced during procedures.

5. When preparing children for procedures, the nurse must consider what factors to individualize the preparation?

    a.

    b.

    c.

    d.

    e.

6. T   F   Procedures should be performed in the child's room whenever possible.

7. What four areas of supportive care should the nurse consider before and during a procedure?

    a.

    b.

    c.

    d.

8. Therapeutic play can be used as part of nursing care to:

    a.

    b.

    c.

9. Match each common nursing procedure with the play activity that would best prepare the child for the experience.

    a. ____ Injections   1. Blowing bubbles

    b. ____ Ambulation   2. Giving a toddler a push-pull toy

    c. ____ Deep breathing   3. Letting child handle syringe, vial, and giving
                                                  injection to a doll
    d. ____ Increasing fluid intake
                                                 4. Cutting gelatin into fun shapes

10. T   F   Parents' presence during anesthesia induction prior to surgery has now become a recommended approach to decrease the anxiety of the child.

11. Research indicates that a child may receive clear liquids up to _____ hours before surgery without risk for aspiration.

12. Numerous preanesthetic drugs are used with children. Drugs used should achieve five goals:

    a.

    b.

    c.

    d.

    e.

13. The definition of *compliance* is:

14. When assessing compliance, the nurse would use the following measurement techniques:

    a.

    b.

    c.

    d.

    e.

    f.

    g.

15. Strategies to enhance compliance are grouped into what four categories?

    a.

    b.

    c.

    d.

General Hygiene and Care

16. Staging of pressure ulcers is used to classify the _____ of _____ _____ that has occurred.

17. To care for their hair properly, African-American children need to have a comb with _____

    _____ _____ and a jar of _____.

18. If diarrhea is present, high-carbohydrate liquids are _____ because they may aggravate the

    diarrhea by an _____ effect.

19. List indications of lack of readiness to advance the diet.

    a.

    b.

    c.

    d.

    e.

20. One of the most common symptoms of illness in children is an _____ _____.

21. Match each term regarding body temperature with its definition.

    a. ____ Set point

    b. ____ Fever

    c. ____ Hyperthermia

    1. An elevation in set point such that body temperature is regulated at a higher level

    2. Occurs when body temperature exceeds set point

    3. The temperature around which body temperature is regulated

22. In treating fever, the most effective intervention is the use of _____ to lower the set point.

23. _____ is the most effective antipyretic when administered as recommended.

24. Are the following statements regarding elevated temperature correct (C) or incorrect (I)?

    a. ____ Environmental measures to reduce fever may be used if tolerated by the child and if they do not induce shivering.

    b. ____ Children's Motrin and Children's Advil are approved for fever reduction in children less than 6 months of age.

    c. ____ Tepid baths or sponging are ineffective in treating febrile children.

    d. ____ Antipyretics are of no value in hyperthermia.

    e. ____ Tepid water baths are not effective in hyperthermia.

Safety

25. Define the following terms related to infection control.

    a. Standard precautions

b. Transmission-based precautions

26. The three types of transmission-based precautions are _____, _____, and

_____ precautions.

27. _____ is the most critical infection-control practice.

28. Discipline is necessary to ensure a child's safety in the hospital. A useful discipline technique is the

_____-_____.

29. The method of transporting children safely is determined by their _____, _____,

and _____.

30. _____ are never used as punishment or as a substitute for observation by nursing staff and

need a _____ order before application.

Collection of Specimens

31. Urine obtained from disposable diapers can be tested accurately for:

32. _____ is used to obtain a sterile urine specimen and is performed using

_____ technique.

33. The most serious complication of collecting a blood specimen by puncturing the heel of the infant is

_____ _____.

Administration of Medication

34. The method most used to determine accurate drug dosage for a child is _____

_____.

35. What are the preferred sites for intramuscular injections in infants and small children?

a.

b.

36. The use of the dorsogluteal site for intramuscular injection is delayed until after the child has been

_____ for a minimum of _____ year(s).

37. What are the factors the nurse must consider when administering intravenous drugs to infants and children?

    a.

    b.

    c.

    d.

    e.

    f.

    g.

    h.

38. _____ _____ _____ _____ are used for intermittent infusion of medication into a peripheral venous route.

39. Identify the types of central venous access devices currently available.

    a.

    b.

    c.

Procedures Related to Maintaining Fluid Balance

40. In order to measure urine loss, diapers can be _____. _____ gram equals _____ ml of urine.

41. The goal of IV therapy is to deliver the prescribed _____ or medications without

    _____.

42. Intravenous infusion pumps are widely used in pediatrics because:

Procedures for Maintaining Respiratory Function

43. The organs most vulnerable to damage from excessive oxygenation (oxygen toxicity) are the

    _____ and the _____.

44. Noninvasive methods of determining oxygen saturation are:

    a.

    b.

45. List the advantages of administering medication by aerosol therapy.

   a.

   b.

   c.

46. T   F   Bronchial drainage is more effective immediately after aerosol therapy.

47. CPT =

48. Air or gas delivered directly to the trachea must be _____.

49. Signs of impending mucus occlusion of a tracheostomy are:

50. How often is the tracheostomy suctioned?

Procedures Related to Alternative Feeding Techniques

51. One method used at the bedside to determine nasogastric tube placement is the measurement of _____ of the gastric aspirate.

52. For children who will be on long-term gastrostomy feeding, a skin level device called the _____-_____,

   or _____ _____, or _____ offers several advantages when compared with the conventional gastrostomy tube.

53. Total parenteral nutrition (TPN) involves the IV infusion of highly concentrated solutions of

   _____, _____, and other nutrients.

54. TPN solutions require infusion into a wide-diameter vessel such as the _____

   _____ _____ and _____ or _____

   _____ _____ approached through the external or internal jugular veins.

Procedures Related to Elimination

55. Plain water is not used in an enema for children because, being hypotonic, it can cause:

56. Fleet Enema is not recommended for children. What are the possible complications of this form of enema?

    a.

    b.

57. A major nursing responsibility in the care of ostomies is to protect the _____ _____ from breakdown.

APPLYING CRITICAL THINKING TO NURSING PRACTICE

A. Franklin, age 5 years, is admitted to the unit for surgery.

   1. What patient goals would address the nursing diagnosis of "Risk for injury related to surgical procedure, anesthesia" for Franklin?

      a.

      b.

      c.

      d.

      e.

   2. List interventions that would achieve the goal "Franklin will demonstrate optimum sense of security."

      a.

      b.

      c.

      d.

   3. List evaluative data you would expect to observe if the following nursing goal was accomplished postoperatively: "Will exhibit no evidence of complications."

B. Juan is admitted with a diagnosis of meningitis and has a fever of 103° F.

   1. How and when would you evaluate whether your intervention of administration of an antipyretic is effective?

2. What interventions on the environment will help reduce Juan's fever?

3. To ensure Juan's safety, you would always make sure the _____ _____ are in the "up" position.

C. Maria, age 4 years, is being discharged after hospitalization for pneumonia.

1. What parameters of care would you teach to her parents to enable them to care for Maria at home?

a.

b.

c.

d.

e.

2. What would you tell these parents regarding selection of toys for play?

D. Daniel, age 6 months, is a patient on the pediatric unit. He is admitted to the unit in severe respiratory distress. He is placed in a mist tent in 30% oxygen.

1. List the interventions that can be used to lessen Daniel's fear of the mist tent.

a.

b.

c.

2. What is the rationale for performing chest physiotherapy before meals or 1 to 2 hours after feeding?

3. How would the nurse evaluate whether the chest physiotherapy was successful in removing excess fluid?

E. Rob, age 11 months, is a patient on the pediatric unit. He is admitted to the unit in respiratory failure, and a tracheostomy is performed.

   1. List the nursing interventions used to care for Rob's tracheostomy.

      a.

      b.

      c.

      d.

      e.

      f.

   2. What would the nurse assess in Rob to determine whether his lungs need to be suctioned?

   3. When suctioning Rob's tracheostomy, the nurse would limit the suctioning to three aspirations in one period. What is the underlying rationale for this action?

F. Debra, 1 day old, is admitted to the pediatric floor for medical evaluation. She has a weak suck reflex and cannot drink from a bottle adequately. She is being fed 1 ounce of Enfamil via gavage every 3 hours.

   1. Give a rationale for each of the following interventions the nurse would perform when feeding Debra via gavage.

      a. Insert feeding tube through mouth.

      b. When checking placement of feeding tube, return aspirated contents to stomach.

      c. Secure feeding tube to cheek, not forehead.

d. Flush indwelling feeding tube with 1 ml sterile water.

e. Position Debra on right side or abdomen after feedings.

2. Before inserting formula in the feeding tube, the nurse assesses whether the tube is correctly positioned in the stomach by:

a.

b.

3. What interventions regarding gavage feeding are validated by the following rationales?

a. Refeed to prevent electrolyte imbalance.

b. Ensure that sucking is associated with feeding.

The Child with Respiratory Dysfunction

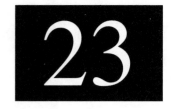

Chapter 23 introduces nursing considerations essential to the care of the child experiencing respiratory dysfunction. The conditions discussed in this chapter impair the exchange of oxygen and/or carbon dioxide and are often more serious in young children. At the completion of this chapter, the student will be able to formulate nursing goals and identify nursing responsibilities to help the child and family effectively cope with the physical, emotional, and psychosocial stressors imposed by an alteration in respiratory function.

REVIEW OF ESSENTIAL CONCEPTS

Respiratory Infection

1. What are the factors that influence the etiology and course of respiratory infections?

    a.

    b.

    c.

    d.

2. Explain why size is a significant variable in respiratory infection of the child.

3. Infants and young children develop generalized signs and symptoms as well as local symptoms when experiencing respiratory infection. Identify the following statements as true or false.

    a. T   F   Newborns may not develop a fever even with severe infections.

    b. T   F   The 6-month-old to 3-year-old will develop fever even with a mild respiratory illness.

    c. T   F   Meningeal signs without infection of the meninges may be present in small children who have an abrupt onset of fever.

    d. T   F   Vomiting is uncommon with respiratory infection.

    e. T   F   Diarrhea may accompany respiratory infection.

    f. T   F   Abdominal pain is an uncommon complaint in small children with a respiratory infection.

    g. T   F   Respiratory illness causes difficulty with feeding because of nasal blockage.

4. What are the nursing goals for the child with an acute respiratory infection and the family?

   a.

   b.

   c.

   d.

   e.

   f.

   g.

   h.

5. _____ _____ _____ may be instilled to clear nasal passages and promote feeding.

Upper Respiratory Tract Infections

6. The therapy for nasopharyngitis is primarily _____.

7. Antihistamines are _____ in treatment of nasopharyngitis.

8. Acute pharyngitis of bacterial origin is usually caused by _____ _____ _____-_____ _____ (_____).

9. A _____ _____ must be done to differentiate between a viral and bacterial throat infection.

10. The recommended treatment for a streptococcal sore throat is:

11. The function of the tonsils is:

12. The _____ _____ are those removed during a tonsillectomy.

13. The pharyngeal tonsils are also known as the _____.

14. The clinical manifestations of tonsillitis are primarily caused by _____. Because of

    swelling, the child has difficulty _____ and _____.

15. Because of the proximity of the adenoids to the posterior nares, swelling causes:

16. The indication for the tonsillectomy and adenoidectomy procedure is controversial. A tonsillectomy is recommended when:

    a.

    b.

    c.

17. Analgesics following a tonsillectomy and adenoidectomy should be administered for at least the first

    _____ _____.

18. The major complication of a T and A is _____.

19. The most obvious sign of bleeding after a T and A is _____ _____ of the trickling blood.

20. Children who have influenza (viral) should not receive _____ because of its link with Reye syndrome.

21. The terminology regarding otitis media is confusing. List the accepted definitions for the following terms.

    a. Otitis media

    b. Acute otitis media

    c. Otitis media with effusion

    d. Chronic otitis media with effusion

22. Acute otitis media is most frequently caused by:

23. In acute otitis media, otoscopy reveals an:

24. When antimicrobial therapy is warranted to treat acute otitis media, the drug of choice for initial treatment

    is _____ _____.

25. Following antibiotic therapy, the child should be evaluated for the effectiveness of the treatment to identify

    the potential complication of _____ _____.

26. During a myringotomy, _____ _____ are used to treat recurrent episodes of
    otitis media with effusion.

Croup Syndromes

27. Croup is usually described or classified according to:

28. The major objectives in medical management of laryngotracheobronchitis (LTB) are:

    a.

    b.

29. Why is the child with LTB placed in an atmosphere of high humidity with cool mist? State the rationale.

30. Acute epiglottitis is:

31. Epiglottitis causes a cherry-red _____ epiglottis.

32. The nurse should not examine the throat of a child with suspected epiglottitis with a tongue depressor
    because:

Infections of the Lower Airway

33. The _____ _____ _____ (_____) is the causative agent of 80
    percent of the cases of bronchiolitis.

34. The primary pathophysiologic process in bronchiolitis that causes difficulty is:

35. The most useful classification of pneumonia is based on the _____ _____.

36. The etiologic agent of pneumonia is identified from:

37. A severe form of atypical pneumonia is _____ _____ _____

_____ (_____).

Other Infections of the Respiratory Tract

38. The causative organism in tuberculosis is _____ _____.

39. The single most important therapeutic modality for TB is _____.

40. What are the three most commonly used drugs to treat TB?

a.

b.

c.

41. The only certain means to prevent tuberculosis is to _____ _____ with the tubercle bacillus.

42. T   F   Bacille Calmette-Guerin (BCG) vaccine is routinely given to treat tuberculosis in the United States.

Pulmonary Dysfunction Caused by Noninfectious Irritants

43. Small children are particularly vulnerable to aspiration of foreign bodies because:

44. Initially, a foreign body in the air passages produces what symptoms?

45. It is the obligation of nurses to learn two simple procedures to treat aspiration of a foreign body. The nurse

should learn and teach the following techniques: _____ _____ and the

_____ _____.

46. The hallmark of ARDS is _____ _____ of the alveolar-capillary membrane, which results in pulmonary edema.

47. Smoke inhalation results in three types of injury. They are:

    a.

    b.

    c.

48. _____ _____ during childhood may be the most important precursor of chronic lung disease in the adult.

Long-Term Respiratory Dysfunction

49. Define *bronchial asthma*.

50. The usual cause of asthmatic manifestations is an:

51. Identify three mechanisms responsible for the obstructive symptoms of asthma.

    a.

    b.

    c.

52. _____ _____ is the central physiologic feature in the clinical manifestations of

    asthma. This forces the individual to breathe at a _____ and _____ lung volume.

53. Children with bronchial asthma exhibit three major symptoms during acute attacks. What are they?

    a.

    b.

    c.

54. The overall goal of asthma management is to _____ _____, to minimize

    _____ and _____ morbidity, and to help the child live as normal and happy a life as possible.

55. _____ control is basic to any therapeutic plan.

56. Early recognition and treatment at the onset of an asthma attack are important. The goal of drug therapy is to:

57. What class of drugs is used to decrease inflammation in asthma?

58. _____ are the major therapeutic agents for the relief of bronchospasm.

59. What are the two types of bronchodilator drugs?

    a.

    b.

60. _____ _____ is an NSAID for asthma.

61. PEFR is _____ _____ _____ _____, measured on the peak expiratory flow meter.

62. Methylxanthines, because of their many side effects, are now _____-_____ agents in the treatment of asthma exacerbations.

63. _____ _____ block inflammatory and bronchospasm effects of leukotrienes.

64. What is the role of exercise in the management of asthma?

65. What components of chest physiotherapy are essential to the management of the asthmatic child?

    a.

    b.

66. The role of hyposensitization in childhood asthma has become _____.

67. Define *status asthmaticus*.

68. The drugs of choice for status asthmaticus are:

69. Children need to be taught the proper use of a _____-_____ _____ with spacer.

70. The principles of self-management of asthma are:

    a.

    b.

    c.

71. Cystic fibrosis is inherited as an:

72. The primary pathologic factor in cystic fibrosis is:

73. The earliest manifestation of cystic fibrosis is _____ _____ in the newborn.

74. Describe the effects of thickened secretions on the gastrointestinal tract of the child with cystic fibrosis.

75. _____ _____ are present in almost all children with cystic fibrosis and constitute the most serious threat to life.

76. Owing to the large amount of undigested food excreted, the stools of the child with cystic fibrosis become:

77. The diagnosis of cystic fibrosis is based on four findings. List them.

    a.

    b.

    c.

    d.

78. A unique diagnostic characteristic of the child with cystic fibrosis is an increased amount of

    _____ and _____ in their sweat.

79. The goals of therapeutic management of the child with cystic fibrosis are:

    a.

    b.

    c.

    d.

80. The goal of pulmonary therapy is:

81. How is the goal of pulmonary therapy met?

    a.

    b.

    c.

82. An aerosolized medication that decreases the viscosity of mucus of the child with cystic fibrosis is

    _____.

83. Pancreatic enzymes are administered to the child with cystic fibrosis according to the following guidelines.

    a. When are they administered?

    b. Dosage depends on:

    c. Amount of enzyme is adjusted to achieve:

84. Children with cystic fibrosis should be placed on a diet that is:

85. The ultimate prognosis for the child with cystic fibrosis is determined by the degree of _____

_____ .

Respiratory Emergency

86. Define the following terms.

    a. Respiratory insufficiency (Describe two types.)

      (1)

      (2)

    b. Respiratory failure

    c. Respiratory arrest

    d. Apnea

87. Cardiac arrest in the pediatric population is usually caused by prolonged _____ rather than cardiac failure.

88. When a child's airway is obstructed, you should attempt to remove the object by:
    a. blind finger sweep of the mouth.
    b. combination of back blows and chest thrusts.

89. The Heimlich maneuver is recommended for children over _____ year(s) of age.

APPLYING CRITICAL THINKING TO NURSING PRACTICE

A. Jackson, age 6 months, is hospitalized with an acute upper respiratory tract infection. He has a fever (104° F), rhinitis, nasal congestion, difficulty feeding, and diarrhea.

    1. List the possible nursing diagnoses for Jackson.

        a.

        b.

        c.

        d.

        e.

        f.

        g.

B. Karen, age 11 months, is seen at the pediatrician's office for a complaint of ear pain and a fever of 102° F. A diagnosis of otitis media is made.

    1. You would intervene with Karen's parents by teaching them the signs of otitis media. List the signs.

    2. List interventions regarding drug therapy that will accomplish the nursing goal "Prevent complications."

C. Peter, age 20 months, is admitted to the pediatric unit with a diagnosis of acute laryngotracheobronchitis. His symptoms on admission include fever, stridor, hoarseness, a brassy cough, dyspnea, irritability, and restlessness.

    1. What would you assess to establish Peter's respiratory status and detect any impending airway obstruction?

    2. Peter's respiratory rate is 70 breaths/minute. Should the nurse encourage fluid intake? If not, what is the underlying rationale?

3. What is the rationale for the use of high humidity with cool mist?

D. Spend a day on a pediatric unit and observe the children admitted for treatment of pneumonia. Differentiate among the various types of pneumonia by completing the following information.

Etiology

1. Viral

2. Primary atypical

3. Bacterial

Therapeutic Management

4. Viral

5. Primary atypical

6. Bacterial

E. Reggie, age 8 years, is admitted to the hospital unit with a diagnosis of suspected tuberculosis.

1. The most important test to establish a diagnosis of tuberculosis is the _____

_____ _____.

2. When teaching Reggie about his drug therapy, the nurse must keep what two principles in mind?

    a.

    b.

3. Reggie's mother asks the nurse whether he can attend school. What should the nurse reply, and what is the rationale?

F. Alice, a 6-year-old white female, came to the emergency room with acute respiratory distress. Her mother noted that she was well until an hour before, when she began to cough without production and "couldn't catch her breath." There is a family history of asthma (her father) and hay fever (her mother).

1. What signs and symptoms of an acute asthmatic attack did you assess in Alice?

2. As the attack progresses, what additional symptoms would you expect to assess?

3. Alice will be treated with a beta-adrenergic agent. Before administering this drug, the nurse should know the intended effects and side effects of the drug.

    a. Intended effects

    b. Side effects

4. What parameters would the nurse assess to recognize status asthmaticus?

5. List the goals that guide the nursing care plan for the child with asthma and the child's family.

    a.

    b.

c.

d.

e.

f.

6. List the expected outcomes for the patient goal "Will exhibit normal respiratory function."

a.

b.

c.

G. Dennis, age 3 years, is hospitalized for treatment of cystic fibrosis.

1. List the possible nursing diagnoses essential to planning the nursing care of Dennis.

a.

b.

c.

d.

e.

f.

g.

h.

i.

j.

2. What are the evaluative data that would give evidence of the attainment of the nursing goal "Help the patient expectorate sputum"?

3. Give a rationale for each of the following clinical manifestations that Dennis displays.

a. Respiratory symptoms

b. Large, bulky, frothy, foul-smelling stools

c. Voracious appetite

d. Weight loss

e. Anemia and bruising

4. Dennis will be going home soon, and his mother must be taught the pulmonary therapy necessary for his care. You would intervene by teaching what three procedures?

a.

b.

c.

The Child with Gastrointestinal Dysfunction

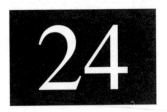

Chapter 24 introduces disorders of the gastrointestinal tract that affect children. These disorders constitute one of the largest categories of illness in infancy and childhood. At the completion of this chapter, the student will be able to assess the child with alteration in gastrointestinal function and will be able to develop goals and responsibilities to help the child and family cope with the stress caused by alteration in gastrointestinal function.

REVIEW OF ESSENTIAL CONCEPTS

Gastrointestinal (GI) Dysfunction

1. Dehydration results when:

2. Infants are prone to disturbance in fluid and electrolytes because they have:
   a. a decreased amount of surface area.
   b. a slower metabolic rate.
   c. a decreased ability to handle solutes and water.
   d. decreased amounts of extracellular fluid.

3. T F   Sodium is the major osmotic force controlling fluid movement.

4. Dehydration is classified as:

5. A sign or symptom that can be present in isotonic dehydration is:
   a. seizures.
   b. serum sodium below 130 mEq/1.
   c. signs of shock.
   d. increased urine output.

Disorders of Motility

6. How is *diarrhea* defined?

7. T F   Chronic diarrhea is often a result of an infectious process.

8. A common clinical manifestation of diarrhea is:
    a. shock.
    b. overhydration.
    c. metabolic alkalosis.
    d. dehydration.

9. Most pathogens that cause diarrhea are spread by the _____-_____ route.

10. The most important viral cause of dehydrating diarrhea in young children is _____.

11. _____ represents 15% of nondysenteric diarrhea in the United States.

12. T   F   Oral rehydration therapy (ORT) is an effective, safer, less painful, and less costly procedure than intravenous rehydration.

13. Signs of dehydration from diarrhea include:

14. Intravenous fluid therapy in mild or moderate diarrhea is directed toward:

    a.

    b.

    c.

15. The best intervention for diarrhea in infants and children is _____.

16. Define *constipation*.

17. _____ _____ is the most common cause of constipation in children between 1 and 3 years of age.

18. The primary defect in congenital aganglionic megacolon is the absence of _____ _____ in one or more segments of the colon.

19. The functional defect in aganglionic megacolon is _____ _____ _____

    _____ (peristalsis) in the affected section of the colon.

20. A _____ _____ is performed to confirm the diagnosis of congenital megacolon.

21. The primary treatment of congenital megacolon is _____ _____.

22. Define *gastroesophageal reflux (GER)*.

23. Although the prone position after feeding is the most effective for infants with GER, this position is contraindicated because of the risk for _____. In children older than one year, it is recommended to use the _____ _____ position with elevation of the _____ _____ _____ _____.

Inflammatory Disorders

24. List the clinical manifestations of appendicitis.

    a.

    b.

    c.

    d.

    e.

    f.

    g.

    h.

    i.

    j.

    k.

    l.

25. The site of most intense pain in appendicitis is _____ _____ located at a point midway between the:

26. T F   Rebound tenderness is a reliable sign of appendicitis in the child.

27. Define *Meckel's diverticulum*.

28. Bleeding can occur in Meckel's diverticulum because:

29. Diagnosis of Meckel's diverticulum is usually based on:

30. Treatment of Meckel's diverticulum is _____ _____.

31. The prognosis is better for which of the inflammatory bowel diseases (IBD)—Crohn disease or ulcerative colitis?

32. The drugs that control the inflammation of IBD are:

    a.

    b.

    c.

    d.

    e.

    f.

33. Is surgical intervention a more effective treatment for Crohn disease or ulcerative colitis?

34. List the clinical manifestations suggestive of peptic ulcer in children over 6 years old.

35. The objectives of therapy for children with peptic ulcers are:

    a.

    b.

    c.

    d.

Hepatic Disorders

36. Hepatitis is caused by at least six types of viruses. List these viruses and their abbreviations.

    a.

    b.

    c.

    d.

    e.

    f.

37. Compare the features of HAV and HBV by completing the following chart.

    Mode of transmission   **Onset**

    a. HAV   c. HAV

    b. HBV   d. HBV

38. Diagnosis of hepatitis is based on:

    a.

    b.

    c.

    d.

39. Identify whether the following statements related to hepatitis A or hepatitis B are true or false.

    a.   T   F   There is no specific treatment for either hepatitis A or hepatitis B.

    b.   T   F   Isolation is required to prevent transmission of the disease.

    c.   T   F   If a patient has had hepatitis A, he or she has crossover immunity to hepatitis B.

    d.   T   F   Immune globulin (IG) is effective in preventing hepatitis A.

    e.   T   F   Handwashing is the single most effective measure in prevention and control of hepatitis.

40. The goals of therapeutic management of cirrhosis are:

    a.

    b.

41. The primary treatment of biliary atresia is _____ _____

    (_____ _____).

Structural Defects

42. The major potential disability for a child with a cleft lip/palate is _____ _____.

43. The immediate nursing problem in the care of the newborn with cleft lip and palate deformities is related to

    _____ the newborn.

44. Clinical manifestations that may indicate the presence of esophageal atresia in a newborn are:

    a.

    b.

    c.

    d.

    e.

45. List the three Cs of a tracheoesophageal fistula.

46. Define *hernia*.

47. A hernia that cannot be reduced easily is called a(n) _____ hernia.

Obstructive Disorders

48. A characteristic symptom of pyloric stenosis is _____ vomiting.

49. Surgical correction of pyloric stenosis is called _____.

50. Define *intussusception*.

51. Definitive diagnosis of intussusception is based on a _____ _____.

52. Abnormal rotation of the intestine around the superior mesenteric artery is called _____. If

    the intestine twists around itself, it is termed _____.

Malabsorption Syndromes

53. _____ _____ is a term applied to disorders characterized by chronic diarrhea
    and malabsorption of nutrients.

54. The classifications of malabsorption syndromes are:

    a.

    b.

    c.

55. The major clinical manifestations of celiac disease are grouped as follows:

    a.

    b.

    c.

    d.

56. Celiac disease may be characterized by acute, severe episodes of profuse, watery diarrhea and vomiting.

    This situation is referred to as a _____ _____.

57. Identify the goals of therapy in short bowel syndrome.

    a.

    b.

    c.

    d.

APPLYING CRITICAL THINKING TO NURSING PRACTICE

A. Valerie, age 2 years, is admitted to the hospital unit with a diagnosis of gastroenteritis due to rotavirus infection.

   1. The major nursing diagnosis for Valerie is:

2. Prevention of the spread of the organism would require which of the following nursing interventions?
    a. Leave diaper open to allow air circulation to skin.
    b. Allow family members to move toys freely from crib to chair and possibly to the home.
    c. Maintain careful handwashing.

3. What evaluative data would reflect the accomplishment of the goal "Skin will remain intact"?

B. Kevin, age 3 years, is brought to the well-child clinic with the complaint of constipation.

1. To help confirm the medical diagnosis of constipation, you would begin your nursing assessment with questions regarding what factors?

    a.

    b.

    c.

    d.

C. Shane, age 11 months, is admitted to the pediatric unit for treatment of Hirschsprung disease.

1. When preparing the parents for the medical treatment Shane will receive for his disease, the nurse would intervene by teaching that the repair of this defect is done in two or three stages. What are they?

    a.

    b.

    c.

D. Stefanie, age 2 months, is admitted for treatment of gastroesophageal reflux (GER).

1. To assist Stefanie to retain feedings, the nurse may advise her mother regarding thickened feedings. What would you teach her?

    a.

    b.

2. The nursing goals for Stefanie are:

    a.

    b.

    c.

E. Tony, age 5 years, is admitted for treatment of appendicitis.

    1. When assessing Tony's pain, the nurse knows that the most reliable estimate of pain is the:

    2. What is the patient goal related to the nursing diagnosis "Risk for spread of infection related to presence of infective organisms in abdomen"?

    3. How will the nurse assess when to request discontinuance of Tony's intermittent gastric decompression?

        a.

        b.

    4. What would be the expected outcome of the patient goal "Will not experience abdominal distention, vomiting"?

F. Spend a day in an ambulatory pediatric clinic. To direct your nursing activities more constructively, differentiate between the two chronic intestinal disorders—ulcerative colitis and Crohn disease—by completing the following information.

Pathologic changes

    1. UC

    2. CD

Rectal bleeding

    3. UC

    4. CD

Diarrhea

  5. UC

  6. CD

Pain

  7. UC

  8. CD

Anorexia

  9. UC

  10. CD

Weight loss

  11. UC

  12. CD

Growth retardation

  13. UC

  14. CD

G. Samuel, age 11 years, is admitted to the pediatric unit with a diagnosis of hepatitis B.

1. Nursing goals for Samuel's care depend on what three factors?

   a.

   b.

   c.

2. The emphasis of nursing care is on encouraging:

H. Care for a child with a cleft lip or palate.

1. Why does feeding pose a special challenge to the nurse?

2. Identify the nursing goals in the postoperative period.

   a.

   b.

   c.

   d.

   e.

3. List evaluation data that would reflect achievement of the goal "No trauma to operative site."

I. Care for a child who has hypertrophic pyloric stenosis.

1. What nursing interventions do you use to achieve the nursing goal of preventing vomiting after surgery?

   a.

   b.

   c.

2. Why is it important for the nurse to monitor hydration status postoperatively?

J.   Jared, age 8 months, is admitted to the emergency room with signs of intermittent abdominal pain, vomiting, and currant-jelly stools. A diagnosis of intussusception is made.

1. As soon as the diagnosis of intussusception is made, the nurse begins to prepare Jared's parents for his immediate hospitalization, the barium enema, and the possibility of surgery. What specific nursing interventions would adequately prepare the parents to deal with each of these stressors?

a. Hospitalization

b. Barium enema

K.   Patricia, age 3 years, is admitted with a diagnosis of celiac disease.

1. A gluten-free diet usually produces dramatic clinical improvement within 2 weeks. Your nursing goal is to teach Patricia and her parents to adhere to this diet. What foods must she avoid?

2. What grains would be included in Patricia's diet?

The Child with Cardiovascular Dysfunction

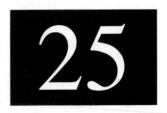

Chapter 25 introduces nursing considerations essential to the care of the child experiencing cardiovascular dysfunction. At the completion of this chapter, the student should have a knowledge of the structural and physiologic changes associated with the various cardiac disorders and will be able to develop appropriate nursing interventions for the child with cardiovascular dysfunction and his family.

REVIEW OF ESSENTIAL CONCEPTS

Cardiovascular Dysfunction

1. A complication that the nurse might assess following a cardiac catheterization is:
   a. hemorrhage at entry site.
   b. rapidly rising blood pressure.
   c. hypostatic pneumonia.
   d. congestive heart failure.

Congenital Heart Disease (CHD)

2. What are the two structures that influence the flow of blood in fetal circulation?

3. T   F   In fetal circulation, the pressure on the left side of the heart exceeds the pressure on the right side.

4. Congenital heart defects are divided into types based on the alterations in circulation. They are

   _____ and _____.

5. An acyanotic heart defect is one in which there is a _____ to _____ shunting of blood.

6. A cyanotic heart defect is one in which there is a _____ to _____ shunting of blood.

7. Another classification system of congenital heart defects is based on hemodynamic characteristics. The four blood flow patterns are:

   a.

   b.

   c.

   d.

8. The classification of acyanotic congenital heart defects is subdivided into the blood flow pattern groups of "increased pulmonary blood flow" and "obstruction to blood flow from ventricles." Match each of the following defects with the appropriate group.

   a. ____ Atrial septal defect (ASD)

   b. ____ Pulmonic stenosis (PS)

   c. ____ Aortic stenosis (AS)

   d. ____ Ventricular septal defect (VSD)

   e. ____ Patent ductus arteriosus (PDA)

   f. ____ Atrioventricular canal (AVC)

   g. ____ Coarctation of the aorta (COA)

   1. Increased pulmonary blood flow

   2. Obstruction to blood flow from ventricles

9. Match the following definitions, clinical manifestations, or treatments with the appropriate congenital cardiac defect. (Not all choices will be used.)

   a. ____ Abnormal opening between the atria, allowing blood from the higher-pressure left atrium to flow to the lower-pressure right atrium

   b. ____ Small defects surgically repaired with a purse-string approach; large defects repaired by a Dacron patch sewn over the opening; both procedures done via cardiopulmonary bypass

   c. ____ Incomplete fusion of endocardial cushions that creates a large central atrioventricular valve, allowing blood to flow between all four chambers of the heart

   d. ____ Has a characteristic machine-like murmur

   e. ____ High blood pressure and bounding pulses in arms; weak or absent femoral pulses; and cool lower extremities with lower blood pressure

   1. Atrial septal defect (ASD)

   2. Pulmonic stenosis (PS)

   3. Patent ductus arteriosus (PDA)

   4. Ventricular septal defect (VSD)

   5. Atrioventricular canal defect (AVC)

   6. Coarctation of the aorta (COA)

   7. Aortic stenosis (AS)

10. The classification of cyanotic congenital heart defects is subdivided into the blood flow pattern groups of "decreased pulmonary blood flow" and "mixed blood flow." Match each of the following defects with the appropriate group.

   a. ____ Tetralogy of Fallot

   b. ____ Tricuspid atresia

   c. ____ Transposition of great arteries

   d. ____ Total anomalous pulmonary venous return

   e. ____ Truncus arteriosus

   f. ____ Hypoplastic left heart syndrome

   1. Decreased pulmonary blood flow

   2. Mixed blood flow

11. Match the following definitions, clinical manifestations, or treatments with the appropriate congenital cardiac defect. (Not all choices will be used.)

a. ____ Classic form includes four defects:
         (1) ventricular septal defect
         (2) pulmonic stenosis
         (3) overriding aorta
         (4) right ventricular hypertrophy

1. Tetralogy of Fallot

2. Tricuspid atresia

b. ____ Treated by arterial switch procedure

3. Transposition of great arteries

4. Total anomalous pulmonary venous return

c. ____ Failure of normal septation and division of the embryonic bulbar trunk into the pulmonary artery and the aorta

5. Truncus arteriosus

6. Hypoplastic left heart syndrome

d. ____ Underdevelopment of left side of heart

Clinical Consequences of Congenital Heart Disease

12. Define *congestive heart failure*.

13. The most common cause of congestive heart failure in children is _____ _____

_____ and _____ within the heart, secondary to structural abnormalities.

14. The two classifications of congestive heart failure are:

a.

b.

15. The signs and symptoms of CHF are divided into three groups. Name them.

a.

b.

c.

16. Related to impaired myocardial functioning, one of the earliest signs of decompensation to assess is

_____.

17. Cardiac failure may lead to pulmonary congestion, producing such signs as:

18. Systemic venous congestion is a primary consequence of right-sided failure and is reflected in the following clinical manifestations:

19. List the four goals of the therapeutic management of congestive heart failure.

    a.

    b.

    c.

    d.

20. Identify the signs of digoxin toxicity in children.

21. Indicate whether the following statements regarding nursing care of the child with a congenital heart disease and congestive heart failure are true or false.

    a.   T   F   The radial pulse is always taken prior to administering digoxin.

    b.   T   F   Feeding is planned to accommodate the infant's sleep and wake patterns.

    c.   T   F   Hypothermia and hyperthermia decrease the need for oxygen.

    d.   T   F   Infants and children should be positioned in at least a 45-degree angle to increase chest expansion.

    e.   T   F   Infants should be fed on a 4-hour schedule in order to decrease fatique.

    f.   T   F   Potassium levels are checked frequently if the child is receiving diuretics.

    g.   T   F   Cyanosis is apparent when oxygen saturation is 80 to 85 percent.

Nursing Care of the Family and Child With Congenital Heart Disease

22. What interventions would the nurse use to help the parents and child adjust to the diagnosis of congenital heart disease?

    a.

    b.

    c.

    d.

    e.

f.

g.

h.

Acquired Cardiovascular Disorders

23. The most common causative agent of bacterial endocarditis is _____

_____.

24. The major sequela to rheumatic fever is heart damage, especially scarring of the _____

_____.

25. Adequate treatment of _____ _____ _____ infection prevents rheumatic fever.

26. Diagnosis of rheumatic fever is based on the presence of two major manifestations or one major and two

minor manifestations as identified by the _____ criteria, in combination with evidence of a recent

_____ infection. The most objective evidence supporting a recent streptococcal infection

is an elevated or rising _____ titer.

27. Define the following terms.

a. Low-density lipoproteins (LDLs)

b. High-density lipoproteins (HDLs)

28. Selected screening techniques for children with high cholesterol levels would target:

29. Dysrhythmias can be classified according to their effect on heart rate and rhythm. List them.

a.

b.

c.

30. Children with sinus bradycardia may need to have a permanent _____ implanted to assist the conduction function of the heart.

31. _____ refers to abnormalities of the myocardium in which the cardiac muscles' ability to contract is impaired.

Heart Transplantation

32. Indications for heart transplantation in children are _____ or _____-_____

_____ _____ _____.

Vascular Dysfunction

33. The diagnosis of hypertension in children and adolescents primarily involves the assessment of the

_____ _____ during every physical examination.

34. Mucocutaneous lymph node syndrome, also known as _____ _____, primarily

affects the _____ system.

35. There is no specific diagnostic laboratory test for Kawasaki disease, so the diagnosis is based on the presence of five of six characteristic symptoms, which must always include an elevated

_____.

36. In the acute stage of Kawasaki disease, nursing interventions include the administration of large doses of

_____ and _____ _____.

37. The physiologic consequences of shock are:

a.

b.

c.

38. The three types of shock are:

a.

b.

c.

39. The three stages or phases of shock are:

a.

b.

c.

40. Identify the three major goals of therapeutic management of shock.

    a.

    b.

    c.

41. Anaphylaxis results from:

42. Identify early cutaneous signs of anaphylaxis.

| **APPLYING CRITICAL THINKING TO NURSING PRACTICE** |

A. Carolyn, 7 years old, is admitted to the pediatric unit for a cardiac catheterization the next morning. She is accompanied by her parents. Both Carolyn and her parents appear anxious. A basic nursing assessment is performed.

    1. The nursing assessment of Carolyn prior to the procedure should include:

    2. Carolyn undergoes her cardiac catheterization and returns to the pediatric unit at noon. She appears drowsy and has a pressure dressing on her right groin area. The most important nursing responsibility associated with the postprocedural care of Carolyn would be the detection of complications. Identify the rationale(s) for each of the following nursing interventions or observations.

       a. Frequent vital signs

       b. Monitor blood pressure, especially for hypotension

       c. Assess pulses distal to the catheterization site

d. Assess the temperature and color of affected extremity

B. Spend a day in an outpatient cardiac clinic to observe the role of the nurse in the management of children with cardiac dysfunction.

1. Identify the factors in a child's history that might be associated with an abnormally high incidence of congenital heart disease.

a. Prenatal factors

b. Genetic factors

2. What clinical manifestations might be seen in a child who is brought to the clinic with a diagnosed ventricular septal defect?

3. A mother is complaining that she has great difficulty feeding her infant with a serous cardiac defect. What interventions would you include to assist her?

C. Care for a hospitalized child with congestive heart failure.

1. Why would a child with congestive heart failure be placed on a regimen of oral digitalis and diuretics?

a. Digitalis

b. Diuretics

2. Since the margin of safety between the therapeutic and toxic dose of digitalis is narrow, the primary goal of the nurse is to prevent digitalis intoxication. What four nursing interventions would accomplish this goal?

   a.

   b.

   c.

   d.

3. What is the primary rationale for the nurse monitoring potassium levels in patients receiving potassium-losing diuretics and digoxin?

4. What signs would the nurse assess to detect digoxin toxicity in children?

5. For each of the following nursing goals, identify at least two appropriate nursing interventions that would be used when caring for a child with congestive heart failure.

   a. Will exhibit improved respiratory function

   b. Will exhibit no additional respiratory or cardiac stress

   c. Will experience reduction of anxiety

   d. Will exhibit no evidence of fluid excess

D. Johnny, age 3 years, is admitted to the pediatric unit with a diagnosis of Kawasaki disease. Upon admission, it is noted that Johnny has a fever of 102.5° F, a diffuse rash particularly evident on his trunk, and an enlargement of the cervical lymph nodes.

1. The six criteria used in establishing a diagnosis of Kawasaki disease are listed below. Develop a nursing diagnosis for each of these criteria.

   a. Fever for 5 or more days

   b. Bilateral conjunctival infection (inflammation) without exudation

   c. Changes of the mucous membranes of the oral cavity, such as erythema, dryness and fissuring of the lips, oropharyngeal reddening, or "strawberry tongue"

   d. Changes in extremities, such as peripheral edema, erythema of palms and soles, periungual disquamation (peeling) of the hands and feet

   e. Polymorphous rash

   f. Cervical lymphadenopathy

2. For each of the following nursing goals, identify at least four appropriate nursing interventions to be used when caring for Johnny.

   a. Control fever

   b. Prevent dehydration

   c. Minimize possible cardiac complications

E. Rose, age 10 months, is admitted to the pediatric unit for surgery to correct a tetralogy of Fallot. She is cyanotic, short of breath, fatigues easily, and is less than 5 percent on her growth chart. Both her parents are present.

1. When the nurse is developing a care plan for Rose, what goals would guide her nursing care?

a.

b.

c.

d.

e.

f.

g.

2. How would you help this family to decrease fear and anxiety and increase coping behaviors?

3. Rose's parents are concerned about her being in pain after surgery. How could the nurse allay their concerns?

The Child with Hematologic or Immunologic Dysfunction

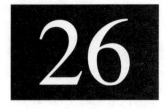

Chapter 26 introduces nursing considerations essential to the care of the child experiencing a dysfunction of the blood or blood-forming organs. A portion of the chapter deals with the hematologic system and its function and provides an overview of the hematopoietic process and the function of the various blood cells. The disorders discussed in this chapter are inherited, chronic, or terminal in nature and result in widespread systemic and structural responses within the body. Upon completion of this chapter, the student will be able to formulate nursing goals and identify the responsibilities that would assist the child and family in adjusting to a hematologic disorder and to prevent or cope with the resulting complications.

REVIEW OF ESSENTIAL CONCEPTS

Hematologic/Immunologic Dysfunction

1. List the components of the complete blood count (CBC).

    a.

    b.

    c.

    d.

    e.

    f.

    g.

    h.

    i.

    j.

    k.

2. A term used when describing an abnormal CBC is "_____ ____ ____ _____," which refers to the presence of immature cells in the peripheral blood from hyperfunction of the bone marrow.

3. Anemia is defined as _____ _____ _____ _____ _____ _____, volume, or hemoglobin concentration to below normal levels.

4. Name the two basic categories of anemia and explain them.

    a.

    b.

204

5. What is the basic physiologic defect caused by anemia?

6. To understand the discussion of anemia, the nurse must be familiar with the terminology. Match each of the following terms with its defining characteristic.

   a. ____ Normocytic

   b. ____ Normochromic

   c. ____ Microcytic

   d. ____ Hypochromic

   e. ____ Hemolysis

   f. ____ Intracorpuscular

   g. ____ Extracorpuscular factor

   h. ____ Macrocytic

   1. Larger than normal size red blood cell (RBC)

   2. Conditions outside RBC that cause hemolysis

   3. Defect within RBC

   4. Normal size RBC

   5. Excessive destruction of RBC

   6. Normal color RBC, normal amount of Hgb

   7. RBCs that are pale in color, reduced amount of Hgb

   8. Smaller than normal size RBC

7. To assess and interpret laboratory studies for integration into a patient assessment, the nurse must understand the following laboratory measures. Identify what is measured by each of these tests.

   a. Mean corpuscular volume (MCV)

   b. Mean corpuscular hemoglobin (MCH)

   c. Mean corpuscular hemoglobin concentration (MCHC)

   d. Red blood cell (RBC) count

   e. Hemoglobin (Hgb)

   f. Hematocrit (Hct)

g. Reticulocyte count

h. White blood cell (WBC) count

i. Differential WBC count

j. Platelet count

Red Blood Cell (RBC) Disorders

8. The objectives of medical management are to _____ the anemia by treating the underlying

   cause and to make up for any _____ of blood, blood component, or substance the blood needs
   for normal functioning.

9. The nursing goals for the care of the child with anemia are:

   a.

   b.

   c.

10. Signs of exertion in the anemic child are:

11. _____ is required for the production of hemoglobin.

12. Often a baby with iron deficiency anemia is called a "milk baby." What is the meaning of this term?

13. In formula-fed infants, the best sources of supplemental iron are:

   a.

   b.

14. The side effects of oral iron therapy are:

15. The main nursing goal regarding diet is:

16. When the proper dose of supplemental iron is reached, the stools usually turn a _____ _____

    _____.

17. Define the following forms of sickle cell disease.

    a. Sickle cell trait

    b. Sickle cell anemia

18. The basic defect in sickle cell anemia is that the red blood cell changes into a _____-

    _____ red blood cell.

19. The basic pathophysiologic changes from sickle cell anemia are primarily the result of:

    a.

    b.

20. List the effects of sickling and infarction on organ structures.

    a.

    b.

    c.

21. The four types of sickle cell crisis are:

    a.

    b.

    c.

    d.

22. Because early identification of sickle cell anemia is essential, the _____ test is used for screening and case-finding.

23. The goals of medical management are:

    a.

    b.

    c.

    d.

    e.

    f.

24. Can oxygen administration reverse sickling of red blood cells?

25. What is the possible negative effect of prolonged oxygen administration for the sickle cell patient?

26. _____ is not used to manage pain in sickle cell patients because it causes seizures in the sickle cell patient.

27. Thalassemia major, or _____ _____, is a severe anemia that is not

    _____ with life without transfusion support.

28. If you trace the pathologic process of thalassemia major, you will see the following sequence: There is

    defective hemoglobin formation; when this formation disintegrates, it causes damage to the _____

    _____ _____, which causes severe _____. To compensate for the hemolytic process, the
    bone marrow produces large numbers of red blood cells. The increase in iron from rapid hemolysis of RBCs

    is stored in various organs. This process is called _____.

29. _____, an iron-chelating agent, is given to the child with thalassemia to minimize the
    development of hemosiderosis.

30. Aplastic anemia has two etiologies. Name them.

    a.

    b.

31. The preferred treatment for aplastic anemia is _____ _____ and/or

    _____ _____ _____.

Defects in Hemostasis

32. Define *hemophilia*.

33. The two most common forms of hemophilia are classic hemophilia and Christmas disease. _____

    _____ accounts for 80–85 percent of all cases of hemophilia. What factors are defective in each
    form?

    a. Classic hemophilia

    b. Christmas disease

34. Hemophilia is transmitted as an ___-_____ _____ _____. The most common
    pattern of transmission is between a carrier female and a son.

35. The most frequent site of bleeding is into the _____ _____.

36. The primary therapy for the hemophiliac is replacement of the _____ _____

    _____.

37. _____ _____ _____ and _____ (_____) are
    the preferred drugs for the child with hemophilia A.

38. Nonsteroidal antiinflammatory drugs (NSAIDs) _____ (should/should not) be used to treat

    joints in the child with hemophilia because they _____ platelet function.

39. Hemophiliacs treated with factor replacement between 1979 and 1985 were exposed to _____.

40. Thrombocytopenic purpura is characterized by:

    a.

    b.

41. In ITP, the platelet count is less than _____. Treatment is primarily _____.

42. T   F   Disseminated intravascular coagulation is a primary disease.

43. To avoid aspiration of blood when a child has an epistaxis, you would tell the child to assume what body position?

Neoplastic Disorders

44. List the two major types of leukemia.

    a.

    b.

45. The two basic pathologic factors that occur in leukemia are:

    a.

    b.

46. List the four main consequences of bone marrow dysfunction.

    a.

    b.

    c.

    d.

47. The clinical manifestations that result from the bone marrow dysfunction are:

48. Definitive diagnosis of leukemia is based on:

49. List the phases of chemotherapeutic therapy for leukemia.

    a.

    b.

    c.

    d.

50. Intrathecal chemotherapy is prophylactic therapy directed toward what anatomic area that is protected from systemic chemotherapy?

51. What are the most common drugs and other therapies used in each of the phases of chemotherapy?
    a. Induction/remission
    b. CNS prophylactic
    c. Intensification/consolidation
    d. Maintenance

52. The most important prognostic factors in determining long-term survival for children with ALL are:

53. Differentiate between Hodgkin disease and non-Hodgkin lymphoma.

    a. Hodgkin disease

    b. Non-Hodgkin lymphoma

54. The primary modalities of therapy for Hodgkin disease are _____ and

    _____, used alone or in combination.

Immunologic Deficiency Disorders

55. The human immunodeficiency virus (HIV) is transmitted by:

56. Children acquire HIV by what three pathways?

    a.

    b.

    c.

57. Nursing considerations are primarily directed at:

58. What is the etiology, therapeutic management, and prognosis of AIDS?

    a. Etiology

    b. Therapeutic management

    c. Prognosis

59. Define *severe combined immunodeficiency disease (SCID)*.

60. The only definitive treatment of SCID is:

61. Wiskott-Aldrich syndrome is characterized by three abnormalities. List them.

    a.

    b.

    c.

Technologic Management of Hematologic/Immunologic Disorders

62. List the major categories of immediate reactions to a blood transfusion.

    a.

    b.

    c.

d.

e.

f.

g.

63. The types of hematopoietic stem cell transplants are:

a.

b.

c.

d.

64. Define the term *apheresis*.

APPLYING CRITICAL THINKING TO NURSING PRACTICE

A. Regina, age 4 years, is admitted to the pediatric unit for diagnosis and treatment of possible anemia.

1. Regina will be undergoing a battery of blood tests. The nursing goal of preparing the child for these tests can be accomplished by what nursing interventions?

a.

b.

c.

2. What nursing diagnoses are appropriate for Regina?

a.

b.

c.

B. Tonisha, age 3 years, is hospitalized with sickle cell anemia.

1. Tonisha has lapsed into a vasoocclusive sickle cell crisis. What nursing diagnoses are appropriate for Tonisha?

a.

b.

2. Management of pain during a sickle cell crisis is a difficult problem. How would you medicate Tonisha to avoid "clock watching" and undermedication?

3. The parents of Tonisha are worried about addiction to pain medicine. What would you say to them?

C. Ryan, age 3 years, is hospitalized for treatment of his hemophilia A.

1. What emergency measures (interventions) could the family institute for a bleeding episode in addition to factor replacement?

a.

b.

c.

d.

2. What measures would the nurse institute to prevent oral bleeding?

D. Billy, age 7 years, is hospitalized with a diagnosis of leukemia.

1. List the patient goals appropriate for the nursing diagnosis "Risk for injury related to interference with cell proliferation."

a.

b.

c.

2. List nursing interventions appropriate to achieve the goal "Will maintain skin integrity."

a.

b.

c.

3. What are the rationales for each of the nursing interventions identified in question 2?

a.

b.

c.

E. Tony, age 4 months, is being treated for AIDS.

1. One of the patient goals for Tony is "Will not spread disease to others." List the interventions that would accomplish this goal.

   a.

   b.

   c.

   d.

   e.

   f.

2. List the nursing diagnoses for Tony and his family.

   a.

   b.

   c.

   d.

   e.

   f.

   g.

The Child with Genitourinary Dysfunction

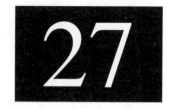

Chapter 27 introduces the nursing considerations essential to the care of the child who is experiencing renal dysfunction. At the completion of this chapter, the student will understand the tests used to assess renal function, the more common disorders of renal function, the various types of dialysis, and renal transplantation. The student will use this knowledge to formulate a nursing care plan for the child and family experiencing renal dysfunction.

REVIEW OF ESSENTIAL CONCEPTS

Genitourinary Dysfunction

1. The single most important diagnostic laboratory test to detect renal problems is the

   _____.

2. The collection of specimens and the performance of screening tests are the nurse's responsibility. Match each of the following tests with its purpose or significance of deviation.

   a. ____ Urinary tract inflammatory process

   b. ____ Specific gravity

   c. ____ Urine culture and sensitivity

   d. ____ Appearance

   e. ____ pH

   1. Determines presence of pathogens and the drugs to which they are sensitive

   2. Normal result: 1.016–1.022; reflects state of hydration

   3. Normal result of urine: 4.8–7.8

   4. Presence of more than 5 polymorphonuclear leukocytes

   5. Normal result: clear, pale yellow to deep gold

Genitourinary Tract Disorders/Defects

3. The single most important host factor influencing the occurrence of a urinary tract infection (UTI) is

   _____   _____.

4. T   F   The presence of alkaline urine inhibits the growth of bacteria.

5. UTIs are often undetected in children. The nurse would suspect a UTI if the child exhibits:

   a.

   b.

   c.

6. List the four objectives of the therapeutic management of the child with a urinary tract infection.

   a.

   b.

   c.

   d.

7. Define *vesicoureteral reflux (VUR)*.

8. Obstruction of the urinary system can be:

   a.

   b.

   c.

   d.

9. Define the following genitourinary anomalies.

   a. Hydronephrosis

   b. Hydrocele

   c. Epispadias

   d. Phimosis

   e. Cryptorchidism

Glomerular Disease

10. The massive edema seen in minimal-change nephrotic syndrome (MCNS) is a result of:
    a. inability to excrete excess sodium.
    b. hypoalbuminemia, leading to decreases in osmotic pressure.
    c. narrowing of the renal afferent arterioles.
    d. decreased urine output, leading to increased intravascular volume.

11. A clinical manifestation of minimal-change nephrotic syndrome is:
    a. hypertension.
    b. coffee-colored urine.
    c. proteinuria.
    d. low specific gravity.

12. _____ are the primary therapeutic agents used to treat MCNS.

13. A side effect of steroid therapy in children is:
    a. growth retardation.
    b. hypotension.
    c. renal calculi.
    d. constipation.

14. Match each clinical manifestation with the renal disease in which it is seen.

    a. ___   Hypertension   1. Nephrotic syndrome

    b. ___   Hematuria   2. Acute glomerulonephritis

    c. ___   Ascites

    d. ___   Azotemia

    e. ___   Increased serum lipid levels

15. List the methods used in the diagnostic evaluation of acute glomerulonephritis.

    a.

    b.

    c.

    d.

    e.

    f.

16. T   F   Monitoring of fluid intake is not required in children with acute glomerulonephritis.

17. T   F   Hypertension is a common result of glomerulonephritis.

18. The function of the _____ _____ is the reabsorption of substances; the function of

    the _____ is filtration.

19. T   F   Urinary tract infections are commonly seen in patients with obstructive uropathy.

Miscellaneous Renal Disorders

20. _____ _____ _____ represents one of the most frequent causes of acquired acute renal failure in childhood.

21. The primary site of injury in hemolytic uremic syndrome is:

22. List the clinical manifestations of hemolytic uremic syndrome.

    a.

    b.

    c.

    d.

    e.

    f.

    g.

    h.

23. The anemia seen in hemolytic uremic syndrome results from:

24. _____ _____ is the most common malignant renal and intraabdominal tumor of childhood.

25. Wilms tumor is treated by combined treatment of _____ and _____ with or without _____, depending on clinical stage and histologic pattern.

26. _____ is indicated for all clinical stages of Wilms tumor.

Renal Failure

27. A most common cause of acute renal failure in children is:
    a. renal hypoplasia.
    b. Alport syndrome.
    c. severe dehydration.
    d. obstructive uropathy.

28. The prime clinical manifestation of acute renal failure is _____.

29. Treatment of acute renal failure is directed toward:

    a.

    b.

    c.

30. Two life-threatening complications of acute renal failure are:

31. T   F   Growth failure is one of the major consequences of chronic renal failure.

Technologic Management of Renal Failure

32. Dialysis is:

33. The types of dialysis are:

    a.

    b.

    c.

34. Which type of dialysis is preferred in order to preserve the child's independence?

35. When renal function is severely compromised, _____ _____ is an acceptable and effective means of therapy in the pediatric age group.

APPLYING CRITICAL THINKING TO NURSING PRACTICE

A. Barry, age 3 months, is brought to the pediatrician by his mother, who says that for the past few days Barry has been eating poorly, is running a high temperature, is sleeping much more than usual, and seems to be voiding large amounts. A urine culture is obtained. The pediatrician believes that Barry may have a urinary tract infection, secondary to an obstruction, and admits him to the hospital.

1. The nursing assessment yielded several signs and symptoms of renal disease in Barry. List them.

    a.

    b.

    c.

2. Why did the pediatrician suspect that Barry may have obstructive uropathy?

3. The most important nursing goal when caring for children with urinary tract infections is

   _____.

4. List the nursing interventions used to care for Barry.

   a.

   b.

   c.

   d.

   e.

   f.

   g.

   h.

B. Care for a child who has minimal-change nephrotic syndrome.

   1. Formulate one nursing diagnosis related to the presence of edema in this child.

   2. List one nursing goal related to the susceptibility of this child to infection.

   3. What is the rationale for providing meticulous skin care?

   4. It is essential to monitor protein levels in the urine. It is difficult to obtain specimens from absorbent disposable diapers. How would you collect the needed specimen without resorting to collection devices that must be taped to edematous skin?

C. Tina, age 6 years, is admitted to the pediatric unit. Tina's history reveals that she had a severe sore throat and had been receiving antibiotics. Her mother stopped giving them when Tina felt better. Her admitting diagnosis is acute glomerulonephritis. She is anuric and has severe hypertension. It is believed that she has acute renal failure, secondary to the nephritis.

1. What nursing intervention might have prevented the occurrence of acute glomerulonephritis in Tina?

2. List the nursing interventions necessary to maintain fluid balance in Tina while she has acute renal failure.

   a.

   b.

   c.

   d.

   e.

   f.

3. In preparation for home care, the parents must be instructed regarding general measures, diet, activity restriction, and prevention of infection. How would the nurse evaluate whether the parents understood her instructions?

D. Betsy is a patient on the pediatric unit. She was first admitted to the unit with hemolytic uremic syndrome. She has recovered from the primary disease but now appears to have chronic renal failure. She is to be taught how to perform home peritoneal dialysis.

1. What were the signs and symptoms of hemolytic uremic syndrome that Betsy probably exhibited?

2. In order for the family to maintain home dialysis, the nurse must teach the family. What areas would be included in this teaching plan?

   a.

   b.

   c.

3. Identify one nursing goal for Betsy related to diet.

4. List the patient goal that will address the nursing diagnosis "Risk for injury related to accumulated electrolytes and waste products."

5. How would you evaluate whether nursing interventions were successful in assisting the child with the stresses of chronic renal failure?

E.   Richard, age 3 years, is admitted for treatment of a Wilms tumor.

1. Because surgery is performed within 24 to 48 hours after admission, the nurse must prepare Richard's parents for this procedure. List at least one nursing intervention to accomplish this.

   a.

   b.

2. Because Richard is prone to intestinal obstruction, what postoperative nursing interventions are appropriate?

   a.

   b.

   c.

   d.

The Child with
Cerebral Dysfunction

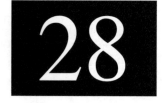

Chapter 28 introduces the nursing considerations essential to the care of the child experiencing cerebral dysfunction. Since the brain is the center for multiple vital body functions, any disturbance in this regulating, controlling, and communicating mechanism can produce alterations in the way in which the system receives, integrates, and responds to stimuli entering the system. Since an alteration in the level of consciousness is a common finding in many cerebral disturbances, the student will be introduced to methods used to assess and diagnose neurologic function in the unconscious child. At the completion of this chapter, the student will be able to develop nursing goals and responsibilities that help the child and family to effectively cope with the multiple stressors imposed by an alteration in cerebral function.

REVIEW OF ESSENTIAL CONCEPTS

Cerebral Dysfunction

1. Because it is difficult to assess cerebral function in the infant and small child, what methods are employed?

   a.

   b.

   c.

   d.

2. List the aspects of assessment for cerebral dysfunction.

   a.

   b.

   c.

3. The early signs and symptoms of increased intracranial pressure are subtle and assume many patterns. List these signs and symptoms for the younger and older child.

   a. Younger child

   b. Older child

4. As intracranial pressure becomes progressively worse, what signs would you expect to assess?

5. List and define the two components of consciousness and explain them.

   a.

   b.

6. Level of consciousness (LOC) is determined primarily by:

7. Match the following terms that describe levels of consciousness with their defining characteristics.

   a. ___ Disorientation

   b. ___ Persistent vegetative state (PVS)

   c. ___ Full consciousness

   d. ___ Obtundation

   e. ___ Confusion

   f. ___ Coma

   g. ___ Stupor

   h. ___ Lethargy

   1. Awake and alert; orientated to time, place, and person

   2. Impaired decision making

   3. Disorientation to time and place; decreased level of consciousness

   4. Limited spontaneous movement; sluggish speech

   5. Arousable with stimulation

   6. Remains in a deep sleep; responsive only to vigorous and repeated stimulation

   7. No motor or verbal response to noxious (painful) stimuli

   8. Function of the cerebral cortex permanently lost

8. The Glasgow Coma Scale (GCS) consists of what three areas of assessment?

   a.

   b.

   c.

9. The purpose of the neurologic examination is to:

10. What areas are assessed in performing a neurologic examination?

11. The sudden appearance of a fixed and dilated pupil is an _____.

12. Define the following terms of posturing.

    a. Decorticate posturing

    b. Decerebrate posturing

13. List the diagnostic procedures, other than blood tests, that are used to assess cerebral function.

    a.

    b.

    c.

    d.

    e.

    f.

    g.

    h.

    i.

    j.

    k.

    l.

    m.

Nursing Care of the Unconscious Child

14. One of the primary concerns when caring for an unconscious patient is to maintain a

    _____ _____.

15. Four major types of ICP monitors are:

    a.

    b.

    c.

    d.

Cerebral Trauma

16. Define the following terms unique to head injuries.

    a. Coup

    b. Contrecoup

17. List and define the types of head injuries.

    a.

    b.

    c.

18. Identify the major complications of trauma to the head.

19. Vascular rupture may occur even in minor head injuries, causing hemorrhage between the skull and cerebral surfaces. Why is the accumulation of blood between the skull and cerebral surfaces dangerous?

20. When bleeding occurs between the skull and cerebral surfaces, the accumulation of blood is called a

    _____.

21. A subdural hemorrhage is bleeding between the _____ and the _____, usually as a

    result of rupture of the _____ _____.

22. Another major complication of head trauma is _____ edema.

23. If cerebral edema is not detected and relieved, what is the consequence to the brain tissue?

24. What diagnostic test is essential in diagnosing neurologic trauma?

25. The most important nursing consideration in caring for a child with a head injury is:

26. The major pulmonary changes that occur in drowning are directly related to:

27. The major problems caused by near-drowning are:

    a.

    b.

    c.

28. Most drownings of children can be _____ with adequate supervision.

Nervous System Tumors

29. The majority of brain tumors in childhood are _____. The other tumors are

    _____.

30. Because the signs and symptoms of brain tumors are related to increasing intracranial pressure, infants with brain tumors do not display easily detectable symptoms. Why not?

31. The most common diagnostic procedure for a brain tumor is _____

    _____ _____ (_____).

32. The treatment of choice for brain tumors is total _____.

33. When the temperature is elevated in a patient after removal of a brain tumor, the nurse would suspect an

    _____ _____.

34. Headache may be severe after surgery in the patient with a brain tumor. The headaches are largely caused by

    _____ _____.

35. The primary site for a neuroblastoma is within the _____ _____ or

    _____ _____ _____.

36. Diagnostic evaluation of neuroblastoma is aimed at locating the _____ _____ and

    _____ ____ _____ _____.

37. Urinary excretion of _____ is detected in approximately 95 percent of children with
    adrenal or sympathetic tumors.

38. Identify the three methods employed to treat neuroblastoma.

39. Neuroblastoma is one of the few tumors that demonstrate a spontaneous _____.

Intracranial Infections

40. Intracranial infections cause inflammation. What three structures can the inflammatory process affect? For
    each of these structures, give the name of the alteration.

    a.

    b.

    c.

41. Haemophilus influenzae type B is prevented by the _____ vaccine.

42. What organisms are responsible for 95 percent of the cases of bacterial meningitis in children older than 2
    months?

    a.

    b.

43. What form of meningitis is readily transmitted to others and by what vehicle?

44. Identify the following statements regarding bacterial meningitis as true or false.

    a.   T   F   Isolation is not needed for bacterial meningitis.

    b.   T   F   Seizures do not occur in affected children.

    c.   T   F   There are no vaccines for bacterial meningitis.

45. The treatment of aseptic meningitis is primarily _____.

46. Encephalitis can occur as a result of:

    a.

    b.

47. Reye syndrome usually follows a common viral illness such as _____ or

    _____.

48. Research has confirmed an association between the use of _____ and the incidence of Reye syndrome.

49. What are the dominant clinical manifestations of human immunodeficiency virus encephalopathy?

50. What are the two types of immunizing products available for rabies in humans?

    a.

    b.

Seizure Disorders

51. The basic mechanism that causes seizures is:

52. What are the two major categories of seizures?

53. Psychomotor seizures are characterized by:

54. The _____ (_____) is one of the most useful diagnostic tools for evaluating seizure disorders.

55. What are the goals of therapeutic management of seizures?

    a.

    b.

    c.

56. What is the action of anticonvulsive drugs?

57. How is the dosage of anticonvulsant drugs monitored?

58. What precautions should be taken if the anticonvulsive drug is discontinued?

59. Tonic-clonic seizures are also known as _____ _____ and _____ seizures.

60. The generalized seizure that is characterized by a brief loss of consciousness with minimal or no alteration in muscle tone and that may go unrecognized is called a _____ _____ or _____ seizure.

61. Define *status epilepticus*.

62. Seizure precautions include:

63. Define *febrile seizures*.

Cerebral Malformations

64. The majority of infants with craniosynostosis have _____ brain development.

65. _____ is a condition caused by an imbalance in the production and absorption of cerebrospinal fluid in the ventricular system, usually under increased pressure.

66. Although the causes of hydrocephalus are varied, the result is either:

    a.

    b.

67. The most commonly observed clinical manifestations of hydrocephalus in the infant include:

    a.

    b.

    c.

    d.

    e.

    f.

    g.

    h.

    i.

68. T   F   The signs and symptoms of hydrocephalus in early and late childhood are caused by increased intracranial pressure.

69. The primary diagnostic tools for detecting hydrocephalus are _____ _____ and _____.

70. The treatment of hydrocephalus usually involves placing a shunt to drain cerebrospinal fluid. This shunt is

    called a _____ (_____) shunt.

APPLYING CRITICAL THINKING TO NURSING PRACTICE

A. Beatrice, age 7 years, was admitted to the pediatric unit after sustaining head trauma in an automobile accident. When admitted, she was conscious and complaining that her head hurt.

   1. Beatrice begins to complain of a headache, nausea, and blurred vision. She seems drowsy. What nursing diagnosis would you formulate from this assessment data?

2. Beatrice is becoming increasingly confused and disoriented. She has limited spontaneous movement, and her speech has become slurred. Based on this assessment, what level of consciousness would best describe Beatrice?

B. Greta, age 8 years, has been unconscious for 3 days as a result of head trauma.

1. List at least three nursing goals for the care of Greta.

a.

b.

c.

2. What parameters are assessed to monitor Greta's neurologic status?

3. List nursing interventions that would achieve the patient goal "Will maintain stable ICP."

a.

b.

c.

d.

e.

f.

g.

4. What is the rationale for placing the child on a water-filled mattress?

5. What is the expected outcome for the patient goal "Child will exhibit no evidence of cerebral edema"?

C. Spend a day in an emergency room for pediatric patients. Answer the following questions, and include specifics (examples, responses) to illustrate these concepts.

 1. Robin, age 3 years, sustained head trauma in a fall down some stairs. She is diagnosed as having a subdural hematoma and is admitted to the pediatric unit. Three important nursing observations are frequent examination of:

 2. Tory, age 3 years, comes to the emergency room after being rescued from a swimming pool. After immediate resuscitation of the child to restore oxygen delivery to the cells, the nurse must be concerned about Tory's parents. What nursing interventions would help comfort the parents?

D. Eden, age 10 months, is admitted to the pediatric unit with a diagnosis of meningococcal meningitis.

 1. What clinical manifestations would you expect to assess in Eden?

 2. Identify the major nursing considerations for the care of Eden.

   a.

   b.

   c.

   d.

   e.

   f.

   g.

   h.

E. Anita, age 4 years, was admitted to the pediatric unit for diagnosis and treatment of a seizure disorder.

 1. To assist with Anita's diagnosis, what data should the nurse gather through a nursing history or direct assessment?

   a.

   b.

   c.

d.

e.

f.

g.

2. While you are giving Anita a bath in bed, she begins to have a seizure. How would you intervene to care for Anita and prevent any injury to her?

a.

b.

c.

d.

e.

f.

3. Anita is diagnosed as having tonic-clonic seizures and is placed on Dilantin. The nurse would formulate a teaching plan regarding drug therapy. The teaching plan would include the following points:

a.

b.

c.

d.

e.

f.

g.

h.

F.   Adam, a newborn, is transferred to the pediatric unit for treatment of hydrocephalus.

1. Postoperative nursing interventions for the child with hydrocephalus include:

a.

b.

c.

d.

e.

f.

g.

h.

i.

j.

2. List the evaluative data that would indicate the accomplishment of the following goal: "The family will receive adequate education and emotional support."

The Child with Endocrine Dysfunction

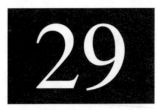

Chapter 29 introduces the nursing considerations essential to the care of the child experiencing endocrine dysfunction. The conditions discussed in this chapter interfere with the body's ability to produce or to respond to the major hormones. The discussion of pancreatic hormone secretion is limited to diabetes mellitus, a relatively common health problem of childhood. At the completion of this chapter, the student will be able to develop nursing goals and responsibilities that will help the child and family develop effective coping responses to deal with endocrine dysfunction.

REVIEW OF ESSENTIAL CONCEPTS

Disorders of Pituitary Function

1. The pituitary gland is also known as the _____ or _____ _____.

2. _____ _____ are the most common cause of pituitary hyposecretion.

3. The main presenting complaint of hypopituitarism is _____ _____.

4. Diagnosis of hypopituitarism is based on absent or subnormal reserves of _____

   _____.

5. The goals of therapeutic management of hypopituitarism are:

   a.

   b.

6. Excess growth hormone before closure of epiphyseal shafts results in proportional _____ ____

   _____ _____; excess after closure of epiphyseal shafts results in _____ ____

   _____ _____, termed _____.

7. Children with a pituitary-secreting tumor may also demonstrate signs of _____

   _____ _____.

8. The primary nursing responsibility regarding hypopituitarism and hyperpituitarism is:

9. The principal disorder of the posterior pituitary hypofunction is _____ _____, which causes hyposecretion of antidiuretic hormone (ADH), producing a state of uncontrolled

   _____.

10. The cardinal signs of diabetes insipidus are _____ and _____.

11. The usual treatment of diabetes insipidus is hormone replacement with _____. The drug

    of choice is _____ _____ (DDAVP).

12. SIADH =

13. SIADH results in:

Disorders of Thyroid Function

14. The _____ gland is the only endocrine gland capable of storing excess amounts of hormones for
    release as needed.

15. The main physiologic action of the thyroid hormone is:

16. The treatment for juvenile hypothyroidism is _____ _____ replacement.

17. A goiter is:

    The synthesis of thyroid hormone depends upon the availability of _____.

18. Graves disease is usually associated with an enlarged _____ _____.

19. List the symptoms that may occur if the patient with thyroid hyperfunction develops thyrotoxicosis.

20. A possible complication of thyroidectomy is _____.

Disorders of Parathyroid Function

21. The objective of therapeutic management of hypoparathyroidism is to maintain normal serum

    _____ and _____ levels with minimum complications.

22. _____ can be secondary to chronic renal disease and congenital anomalies of the uri-
    nary tract.

Disorders of Adrenal Function

23. Identify whether the following hormones are secreted by the adrenal cortex or the adrenal medulla.

    a. ___   Glucocorticoids (cortisol)

    b. ___   Catecholamines (epinephrine)

    c. ___   Catecholamines (norepinephrine)

    d. ___   Mineralocorticoids (aldosterone)

    e. ___   Sex steroids

    1. Adrenal cortex

    2. Adrenal medulla

24. Identify whether the following clinical manifestations are indicative of (1) acute adrenocortical insufficiency or (2) hyperfunction of the adrenal gland (Cushing syndrome).

    a. ___   Increased irritability; headache; diffuse abdominal pain; weakness; nausea and vomiting; diarrhea; fever; and CNS symptoms

    b. ___   Centripetal fat distribution; "moon" face; muscular wasting; thin skin and subcutaneous tissue; poor wound healing; increased susceptibility to infection; decreased inflammatory response; excessive bruising; petechial hemorrhages; facial plethora; reddish purple abdominal striae; hypertension; hypokalemia; alkalosis; osteoporosis; hypercalciuria/renal calculi, psychoses; peptic ulcer; hyperglycemia; virilization; amenorrhea; impotence

25. The administration of excessive amounts of exogenous corticosteroids can result in _____

    _____ _____.

26. A characteristic sign of excess cortisol, whether from exogenous steroid therapy or malfunction of the

    adrenal gland, is the _____ face.

27. Untreated congenital adrenogenital hyperplasia results in early _____ maturation.

28. A sex is assigned to the child with adrenogenital hyperplasia that is consistent with the _____.

29. Urinary levels of 17-ketosteroids are increased in _____ _____.

30. Pheochromocytomas have a familial transmission as an autosomal-_____ trait.

31. The clinical manifestations of pheochromocytoma are caused by _____

    _____ ___ _____.

Disorders of Pancreatic Hormone Function

32. The islets of Langerhans of the pancreas have three major functioning cells. List the hormone produced by each of these cells and its function.

    a. Alpha

b. Beta

c. Delta

33. The two types of diabetes mellitus are:

a.

b.

34. Trace the pathophysiology of diabetes mellitus by describing the etiology underlying each of the following physical consequences.

a. Insulin absence

b. Hyperglycemia

c. Glycosuria

d. Polyuria

e. Polydipsia

f. Metabolism of proteins and fats

g. Glucogenesis

h. Polyphagia

i. Ketonuria and acetone breath

j. Metabolic acidosis

35. What are the long-term complications of diabetes mellitus? (Identify the general type of complication and list three specific examples.)

a.

(1)

(2)

(3)

36. What are the three "polys" of diabetes mellitus?

37. Diagnosis of diabetes mellitus is based on _____ _____ _____.

38. Human insulin is packaged in the strength of 100 units/ml. Match each of the following types of insulin with the appropriate rate of action (peak effect).

a. ____ NPH   1. Rapid-acting

b. ____ Regular insulin   2. Short-acting

c. ____ Lispro insulin   3. Intermediate-acting

d. ____ Ultralente   4. Long-acting

39. _____ _____ are designed to deliver fixed amounts of regular insulin continuously, thereby imitating the release of the hormone by the islet cells.

40. _____-_____ _____ _____ (SBGM) has improved diabetes management and can be used successfully by children.

41. _____ _____ levels are of value in assessing glucose levels over the previous 2 to 3 months. Acceptable levels for children are less than _____.

42. Exercise is beneficial to the child with diabetes because it _____ blood glucose levels.

43. Describe the Somogyi effect.

44. The most common cause of hypoglycemia is _____ _____.

45. Hyperglycemia is also called _____ _____ (DKA).

46. Differentiate between ketoacidosis and a hypoglycemic reaction by completing the following chart.

	Hypoglycemia	Hyperglycemia
Onset	a.	b.
Cause	c.	d.
Manifestations	e.	f.
Ominous features	g.	h.
Urinary findings	i.	j.
Blood glucose	k.	l.

47. The appropriate emergency measure when a child with diabetes is having a hypoglycemic reaction is to

administer _____ in some form.

48. Insulin injections are rotated to various parts of the body. What is the rational for this action?

49. Compliance to the diabetic regimen is sometimes a problem, especially in the _____ age group.

APPLYING CRITICAL THINKING TO NURSING PRACTICE

A. Spend a day in a pediatric endocrine clinic. Answer the following questions, and include specific examples or responses to illustrate these concepts.

1. List the clinical manifestations you would expect to assess in a child with hypopituitarism.

   a.

   b.

   c.

   d.

   e.

   f.

   g.

   h.

   i.

   j.

   k.

2. List the clinical manifestations you would expect to assess in a child with hyperpituitarism before epiphyseal closure.

   a.

   b.

   c.

   d.

3. List the clinical manifestations you would expect to assess in an infant with diabetes insipidus.

   a.

   b.

   c.

   d.

4. What piece of assessment data would alert you to the possibility of an infant having hypothyroidism?

5. The primary nursing goal in relation to hypothyroidism is:

6. List nursing interventions to achieve the following nursing goal in a patient experiencing a deficiency in parathyroid: "Maintain the safety of the patient."

   a.

   b.

   c.

   d.

B. Care for a child with adrenocortical insufficiency. Answer the following questions and include specifics (examples, responses) to illustrate these concepts.

   1. You take the child's vital signs every 15 minutes. What is the rationale for this intervention?

   2. When administering cortisol to the child, you carefully check the dosage and the rate of administration. What is the rationale for these actions?

   3. As treatment progresses, you continually assess the child for signs of hypokalemia. What are these signs?

C. Care for a child with the salt-losing form of congenital adrenogenital hyperplasia.

1. A primary nursing goal in relation to the child with adrenogenital hyperplasia is:

2. The rationale for administering cortisone to the child with adrenogenital syndrome is:

D. Bobby, an 8-year old, is on the pediatric unit for diagnosis and treatment of diabetes mellitus.

1. When Bobby arrived on the unit, he was displaying symptoms of ketoacidosis.

a. What are the four goals for the management of Bobby's care?

(1)

(2)

(3)

(4)

b. List evaluation data you would expect for the nursing goal "Ensure adequate hydration."

2. Bobby is placed on NPH insulin twice per day. The nurse must intervene by monitoring whether the insulin dose is appropriate. What is the best method to do this?

3. Bobby will be maintained on a balanced diet employing the exchange system of the American Diabetic Association. The nursing goal regarding this diet is to:

4. Bobby is experiencing a hypoglycemic reaction.

a. What symptoms would you expect to assess in Bobby?

b. How would you intervene to treat the hypoglycemia?

5. What are the interventions to accomplish the patient goal of "Will demonstrate ability to test blood glucose level"?

a.

b.

c.

6. What is the rational for the intervention "Interpretation of results"?

7. List evaluative data that would indicate the accomplishment of the goal "Child will engage in self-management."

E. Design a teaching plan for the child with diabetes mellitus.

1. What nursing goals are appropriate to include in this teaching plan?

a.

b.

c.

d.

e.

f.

g.

h.

i.

j.

k.

The Child with Integumentary Dysfunction

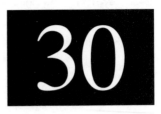

Chapter 30 introduces the various disorders that affect the skin, the largest organ in the body. Alterations in the integrity of the skin by the following causes are explored: bacterial, viral, and fungal infections; environmental and internal antigens; stings and bites; and thermal injury. The knowledge gained in this chapter will help the student formulate an effective care plan for the child with an alteration in skin integrity.

REVIEW OF ESSENTIAL CONCEPTS

Integumentary Dysfunction

1. T   F   The skin is the largest organ in the body.

2. List the four general etiologic factors related to skin lesions.

   a.

   b.

   c.

   d.

3. Match the following terms with the appropriate definitions.

   a. ____ Anesthesia

   b. ____ Paresthesia

   c. ____ Pruritis

   d. ____ Hypesthesia, hypoesthesia

   1. Itching

   2. Alteration in local feeling or sensation, including absence of sensation

   3. Diminished sensation

   4. Abnormal sensation such as burning or prickling

4. Match the following terms used to describe skin lesions with the correct definitions or characteristics.

a. ____ Erythema

b. ____ Ecchymoses

c. ____ Petechiae

d. ____ Primary lesions

e. ____ Secondary lesions

f. ____ Macule

g. ____ Patch

h. ____ Plaque

i. ____ Wheal

1. Tiny pinpoint and sharply circumscribed spots in the superficial layers of the epidermis

2. Localized red or purple discolorations caused by extravasation of blood into the dermis and subcutaneous tissues

3. Changes that result from alteration in a lesion, such as those caused by rubbing

4. A reddened area caused by increased amounts of oxygenated blood in the dermal vasculature

5. Skin changes produced by some causative factor

6. Elevated, flat-topped, and firm; rough, superficial papule greater than 1 cm in diameter

7. Flat, nonpalpable, and irregular in shape; macule greater than 1 cm in diameter

8. Flat, nonpalpable, and circumscribed; less than 1 cm in diameter; brown, red-purple, white, tan

9. Elevated, irregular-shaped area of cutaneous edema; solid, pale pink with lighter center

5. *Wounds* are defined as:

6. Wounds are classified in the same manner as burns. List those classifications.

a.

b.

c.

7. The mechanism of wound healing with scar formation involves the processes of:

a.

b.

c.

d.

8. The major goals of therapeutic management in wound healing are:

   a.

   b.

   c.

   d.

9. Traditional gauze dressings have been replaced with _____ _____ healing dressings.

10. Application of heat to the skin tends to _____ most conditions.

11. The nurse should teach parents that hydrocortisone preparations:
    a. can be used for all skin disorders.
    b. should be applied as a heavy coating.
    c. should be massaged into the skin in a thin layer.
    d. can be used only for 1 to 2 days.

12. To assist in the diagnosis of a skin disorder, the nurse must assess the character of the skin, using the tech-

    niques of _____ and _____.

13. Signs of wound infection are:

14. The wound bed is assessed for:

15. Most of the therapeutic regimens in caring for disorders of the skin are directed toward relief of

    _____.

16. Wet compresses or dressings fulfill the following therapeutic purposes:

17. When taking a bath, use a solution of _____ or _____ _____ to
    relieve pruritis and inflammation.

Infections of the Skin

18. T   F   The incidence of staphylococcal infections in children increases with advancing age.

19. The two major nursing goals related to bacterial skin infections are:

    a.

    b.

20. When a child is admitted to the hospital with cellulitis, nursing interventions include:

    a.

    b.

21. In what two ways do epidermal cells react to viral infection?

    a.

    b.

22. Dermatophytoses (ringworms) are treated with the drug _____ for a period of weeks or months.

Skin Disorders Related to Chemical or Physical Contacts

23. Define *contact dermatitis*.

24. The major nursing goal in the care of the child with contact dermatitis is to:

25. T   F   A nursing intervention following known contact with a poisonous plant is to immediately help the child scrub the affected area with hot, soapy water.

26. The organ in which adverse drug reactions are most often seen is the:
    a. kidney.
    b. heart.
    c. bone marrow.
    d. skin.

27. Describe the nurse's responsibility when a rash is suspected to represent a drug reaction.

Skin Disorders Related to Insect and Animal Contacts

28. List the four areas of the child's body that the nurse should be particularly careful to assess for scabies lesions.

    a.

    b.

    c.

    d.

29. Scabies is treated by the application of _____.

30. In teaching parents about pediculosis capitis, the nurse should emphasize which of the following?
    a. Head lice are carried by household pets.
    b. Lice can be transmitted on personal items.
    c. Cleanliness is the best protection against lice.
    d. Cutting the child's hair prevents reinfestation.

31. Children who are hypersensitive to insect bites or stings should carry the drug

    _____.

32. The major goal of nursing care for Lyme disease should be:

33. T   F   Cat scratch disease is a benign, self-limiting illness that resolves spontaneously in 2 to 4 months.

Skin Disorders Associated With Specific Age Groups

34. The most common contact dermatitis in infants occurs on the convex surfaces of the diaper area as a result of contact irritation from:

35. The aims of nursing management for diaper dermatitis are to:

    a.

    b.

    c.

36. Match each skin disorder with its clinical manifestations.

    a. ___ Seborrheic dermatitis

    b. ___ Atopic dermatitis (eczema)

    c. ___ Diaper dermatitis

    1. Appears on scalp, face, arms, and legs; lesions are red, have papules and vesicles, and are itchy

    2. Appears on the scalp, eyelids, and external ear canal; lesions are thick, yellowish, and scaly

    3. Appears on convex skin surfaces of buttocks, inner thighs, mons pubis, or scrotum

37. List the goals of therapeutic management of eczema.

a.

b.

c.

d.

38. Two new immunomodulator medications used in children with atopic dermatitis are

_____ and _____.

39. Define *seborrheic dermatitis*.

40. The skin disorder that appears predominantly during the adolescent period is _____

_____.

41. Which statement correctly describes acne?
a. The peak incidence of acne is during the period of middle childhood.
b. Lesions seen in acne may be either noninflamed comedones or inflamed lesions.
c. The pathogenesis of acne is related to an abnormality of the sebaceous glands.
d. Primary inflammation in acne is usually caused by the presence of *Staphylococcus albus*.

42. The most effective topical therapy for acne involves the use of _____ or

_____ _____, or a combination of the two drugs.

43. Acutane is given only for severe cystic acne because of the potentially serious _____

_____.

Thermal Injury

44. What are the factors considered in assessing the severity of a burn?

a.

b.

45. A characteristic of a superficial burn is:
    a. absence of pain.
    b. major tissue damage.
    c. systemic effects.
    d. frequently, a latent period followed by erythema.

46. Why is anemia often seen in patients with a burn injury?

47. The immediate threat to life following a serious thermal injury is _____.

48. The primary concerns of therapeutic management of major burns are:

    a.

    b.

    c.

    d.

49. The objectives of fluid replacement for the child with burns are:

    a.

    b.

    c.

    d.

    e.

    f.

50. The early surgical excision of eschar in deep partial-thickness and full-thickness burns reduces:

51. Differentiate between open and occlusive dressing for burns.

    a. Open

    b. Occlusive

52. A homograft is:

53. The goals of nursing care for the burned child and the family are:

    a.

    b.

    c.

    d.

    e.

    f.

54. What is the major problem as burn wounds heal?

55. _____ from sunburn is the major goal of medical and nursing management.

56. Frostbite results from:

APPLYING CRITICAL THINKING TO NURSING PRACTICE

A. A home visit has been scheduled to assist Mrs. Stone in caring for her 5-month-old infant, Andrew, who has atopic dermatitis.

    1. The nursing objectives for caring for the child with atopic dermatitis (eczema) are:

       a.

       b.

       c.

       d.

    2. Formulate at least three nursing diagnoses that pertain to the child who has eczema.

       a.

       b.

       c.

B. Mrs. Ryan brings 2-month-old Sean to the clinic for his well-child visit. Upon examination, you discover that Sean has severe diaper dermatitis.

1. How was the diagnosis of diaper dermatitis made?

2. Nursing interventions for diaper dermatitis are aimed at altering:

3. What interventions might you suggest to Mrs. Ryan to treat and prevent the diaper rash?

a.

b.

c.

d.

e.

f.

g.

C. Michael, age 9 years, is brought to the pediatric health center by his mother. She states that Michael has been scratching his head and that she has found small white specks in his hair. Michael's mother brings a note from the school stating that head lice have been found in several children in Michael's classroom.

1. Why are schoolchildren highly susceptible to infestations of head lice?

2. What causes the characteristic itching seen with pediculosis?

3. _____ or _____ are the drugs of choice in the treatment of pediculosis.

4. What two types of programs must accompany the treatment of pediculosis for it to be effective?

a.

b.

D. Care for a child who has sustained a thermal injury.

    1. What interventions will achieve the patient goal "Maintain the integrity of the skin graft"?

        a.

        b.

        c.

        d.

        e.

    2. What is the expected outcome of the patient goal "Child will maintain adequate fluid hydration status during the acute postburn period"?

    3. What is the rationale for the intervention "Wearing sterile gowns, masks, and gloves while in the patient's room" (under Nursing Dx. "Risk for infection, etc.")?

    4. You notice that your patient is not eating all of the food on the plate. Formulate one nursing diagnosis that reflects this observation.

    5. What is the rationale for the intervention "Carry out range-of-motion exercises" (under Nursing Dx. "Impaired physical mobility, etc.")?

    6. What would you evaluate (expected outcome) that would indicate the achievement of the goal "Family will be prepared for discharge and home care" (under Nursing Dx. "Interrupted family processes, etc.")?

The Child with Musculoskeletal or Articular Dysfunction

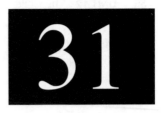

Chapter 31 introduces nursing considerations for the care of the child immobilized with an injury or a degenerative disease. The disorders considered are of congenital, acquired, traumatic, infectious, neoplastic, or idiopathic origin. The conditions may be either temporary or permanent; however, they all affect the child's locomotive ability to a greater or lesser extent. Nursing goals and responsibilities are developed to help the child and family effectively cope with the physical, emotional, and psychosocial stressors imposed by impaired mobility.

REVIEW OF ESSENTIAL CONCEPTS

The Immobilized Child

1. The major physiological effects of immobilization are related directly or indirectly to decreased

   _____ _____.

2. The nurse's physical assessment of the immobilized child focuses not only on the injured part but also on:

Traumatic Injury

3. Define the following traumatic injuries.

   a. Contusion

   b. Dislocation

   c. Sprain

   d. Strain

4. During the first 12 hours of injury, the basic principles of managing soft tissue injuries are represented by RICE. Explain.

   a. R

   b. I

   c. C

   d. E

5. List and describe the most commonly seen types of fractures in children.

   a.

   b.

   c.

   d.

6. The four goals of therapeutic management of fractures are:

   a.

   b.

   c.

   d.

7. In children, the bone fragments are usually treated by being realigned and immobilized by _____

   or by _____ _____ and casting until adequate callus is formed.

8. During the first few hours after a cast is applied, the nurse must observe the cast and the involved extremity for signs of neurovascular integrity. What signs would indicate compromise in the extremity?

9. What are the three primary purposes for use of traction for reduction of fractures?

   a.

   b.

   c.

10. What are the three types of traction?

    a.

    b.

    c.

11. Compare the functions of the various types of traction for the lower extremity by matching the following.

    a. ____ This is a form of running traction in which legs are in an extended position.

    b. ____ This form of skin traction has two lines of pull, one along the longitudinal line of the lower leg and one perpendicular to the leg.

    c. ____ The lower leg is put in a boot cast, and a skeletal Steinmann pin is placed in the distal fragment of the femur.

    d. ____ The leg is suspended in a desired flexed position to relax the hip and hamstring muscles; no traction is exerted directly on a body part.

    1. Balance suspension

    2. 90°-90° traction

    3. Buck's extension

    4. Russell traction

12. When amputated, a severed part should be preserved in what manner to facilitate reattachment?

Congenital Defects

13. List the three degrees of developmental dysplasia of the hip.

    a.

    b.

    c.

14. In the child between birth and 2 months of age, subluxation and the tendency to dislocate are most reliably

    demonstrated by the _____ and _____ tests.

15. Match each type of club foot position with its defining characteristic.

    a. ____ Talipes varus

    b. ____ Talipes equinus

    c. ____ Talipes valgus

    d. ____ Talipes calcaneus

    1. Plantar flexion, in which the toes are lower than the heel

    2. An eversion, or bending outward

    3. Dorsiflexion, in which the toes are higher than the heel

    4. An inversion, or bending inward

16. Therapeutic management of congenital club foot involves:

    a.

    b.

    c.

17. Osteogenesis imperfecta is a group of _____ _____-_____

    _____ characterized by excessive fractures and bone deformity.

Acquired Defects

18. List the four stages of Legg-Calvè-Perthes disease.

    a. Stage I

    b. Stage II

    c. Stage III

    d. Stage IV

19. Define *scoliosis*.

20. Scoliosis is currently managed by the straightening and realignment of the vertebrae by either

    _____ or _____ _____ _____.

21. _____ and _____ are the primary modes of therapy for minor curvatures.

22. The surgical technique consists of realignment and straightening with _____

    _____ and _____ combined with bony fusion of the realigned spine.

23. What is the primary advantage of the L-rod segmental spinal instrumentation method of spinal fusion?

24. Postoperative care following a spinal fusion requires the patient to be _____-_____ when
    changing position to prevent damage to the fusion.

Infections of Bone and Joints

25. Osteomyelitis is an _____ _____ _____ _____, which can be acquired

    from _____ or _____ sources.

26. When the infective agent of osteomyelitis is identified, vigorous _____

_____ is initiated with an appropriate _____.

27. In addition to antibiotic therapy, the child with osteomyelitis is placed on _____ _____, and the

affected extremity is _____.

Bone and Soft Tissue Tumors

28. In children, two types of bone tumors that account for 85 percent of all primary malignant bone tumors are:

29. Compare osteogenic sarcoma and Ewing sarcoma in terms of pathology and therapeutic management.

	Osteosarcoma	**Ewing**
Pathology	a.	b.
Management	c.	d.

30. If an amputation is performed for osteogenic sarcoma, the child may be fitted with a temporary

_____ immediately after surgery.

31. The most common soft tissue sarcoma in children is _____.

32. The most common site for rhabdomyosarcoma is the head and neck, especially the _____.

Disorders of the Joints

33. T   F   There are definitive tests to diagnose juvenile idiopathic arthritis (JIA) in children.

34. What are the major goals of therapy for the child with JIA?

a.

b.

c.

d.

35. The primary groups of drugs prescribed for JIA are:

    a.

    b.

    c.

    d.

36. Why are corticosteroids not the first drugs of choice for JIA?

37. Define *systemic lupus erythematosus (SLE)*.

38. SLE can affect almost any tissue, so the clinical manifestations vary according to the tissue affected. However, a characteristic cutaneous response of SLE is:

39. Identify the goals of therapeutic management of SLE.

    a.

    b.

40. Identify the principal drugs employed to control the inflammation of SLE.

41. Identify the principal nursing goal for the child with SLE.

> ### APPLYING CRITICAL THINKING TO NURSING PRACTICE

A. Spend a day on the neurologic unit observing the care of immobilized children. The nurse must plan the care of the immobilized child with the knowledge that immobilization causes functional and metabolic responses in most of the body systems.

   1. What is the rationale for frequent position changes?

   2. List interventions that would accomplish the patient goal "Child will participate in own care."

     a.

     b.

     c.

     d.

B. Spend a day on a pediatric orthopedic unit.

   1. A 5-year-old child with a fractured right leg has just had a cast applied. The nurse must intervene by teaching the parents how to care for the cast. What elements would you include in your teaching plan regarding methods to decrease the swelling under the cast?

     a.

     b.

     c.

     d.

   2. What elements would you include in a teaching plan regarding maintaining the integrity of the cast?

     a.

     b.

     c.

C. Roger, age 13 years, is in 90°-90° traction for treatment of a fracture of the right femur.

   1. Identify the nursing interventions that will achieve the nursing goal "Maintain the traction."

     a.

     b.

     c.

    d.

    e.

    f.

    g.

2. List interventions that will meet the nursing goal "Maintain alignment."

    a.

    b.

    c.

    d.

D. Care for a child with developmental dysplasia of the hip.

1. During the infant assessment process, what clinical signs could indicate developmental dysplasia of the hip in the newborn?

    a.

    b.

    c.

    d.

    e.

2. Therapeutic treatment is begun as _____ as possible and will vary according to the

   _____ of the child and the extent of the _____.

3. What instructions should be incorporated into a teaching plan for the parents of a child being discharged with a reduction appliance such as a Pavlik harness?

    a.

    b.

    c.

    d.

    e.

E. Jane, age 14 years, is admitted to the adolescent unit with a diagnosis of scoliosis. She is being prepared for an L-rod segmental instrumentation.

1. What are two possible important nursing diagnoses that may be evident when the nurse considers the interaction of Jane's physical defect and psychologic growth and developmental processes of the adolescent?

a.

b.

2. List nursing interventions appropriate to promote the nursing goal "Help the child develop a positive self-image."

a.

b.

c.

d.

3. To control the pain after surgery, what would be the most appropriate choice of drug and method of administration?

F. Emmanuel, age 10 years, is admitted for treatment of osteomyelitis.

1. What clinical manifestations would you expect to assess in Emmanuel if the diagnosis is correct?

2. List nursing interventions appropriate for the nursing goal "Maintain intravenous infusion."

a.

b.

c.

d.

G. Noah, age 11 years, is admitted to the pediatric unit for treatment of JIA.

1. The former drug of choice for treating JIA was aspirin. It has been replaced by what class of drug? Why was aspirin replaced?

2. Identify four nursing diagnoses appropriate for Noah.

    a.

    b.

    c.

    d.

3. List the evaluative data you would observe if the following patient goal was achieved: "Child will be able to be mobile without discomfort."

The Child with Neuromuscular or Muscular Dysfunction

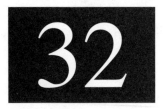

Chapter 32 introduces nursing considerations essential to the care of the child with a disorder of neuromuscular function. The conditions discussed in this chapter may result from defective transmission of nerve impulses to muscles, dysfunction of peripheral motor or sensory nerves, or damage to the central nervous system. At the completion of this chapter, the student will be able to formulate nursing measures directed toward helping the child and family develop effective coping responses to deal with alterations in neuromuscular function.

REVIEW OF ESSENTIAL CONCEPTS

Congenital Neuromuscular or Muscular Disorders

1. Define *cerebral palsy*.

2. Is there a characteristic pathologic picture of cerebral palsy?

3. Classifications of cerebral palsy are based on the nature and distribution of neuromuscular dysfunction. List them.

   a.

   b.

   c.

   d.

4. In order to identify cerebral palsy early in the affected child's life, the nurse would assess what physical warning signs?

   a.

   b.

   c.

   d.

   e.

   f.

5. What is the relationship between cerebral palsy and mental retardation?

6. The broad goals of therapeutic management for the child with cerebral palsy are:

   a.

   b.

   c.

   d.

   e.

7. _____ and _____ are two new drugs utilized to decrease spacticity in the child with cerebral palsy.

8. _____ refers to a hernial protrusion of a saclike cyst containing meninges, spinal fluid, and a portion of the spinal cord with its nerves through a defect in the vertebral column.
   a. Rachischisis
   b. Meningocele
   c. Encephalocele
   d. Myelomeningocele

9. An important nursing intervention when caring for a child with a myelomeningocele in the preoperative stage would be:
   a. applying a heat lamp to facilitate drying and toughening of the sac.
   b. assessing sensory and motor function frequently to monitor for signs of impairment.
   c. applying a diaper to prevent contamination of the sac.
   d. placing the child on his side to decrease pressure on the spinal cord.

10. What are the important goals of therapy regarding latex allergy?

   a.

   b.

11. Define *Werdnig-Hoffmann disease*.

12. All of the muscular dystrophies have a genetic origin in which there is a gradual degeneration of

   _____ _____, and all are characterized by:

13. In all forms of muscular dystrophy, there is insidious loss of strength; the various forms differ in regard to:

14. The most severe and most common muscular dystrophy of childhood is:

15. The cause of death in Duchenne muscular dystrophy is:

16. The primary goals of therapeutic management are:

a.

b.

Acquired Neuromuscular Disorders

17. Guillain-Barrè syndrome is an:

18. Treatment of Guillain-Barrè syndrome is symptomatic and may require _____

_____ to preserve life.

19. Tetanus is:

20. Preventive measures for tetanus are based on the _____ _____ of the affected

child and the nature of the _____.

21. The unimmunized child who sustains a tetanus-prone wound should receive:

22. Infant botulism is caused by:

23. Although inadequately cooked or improperly canned food is the prime source of botulism, the organism has

    been found in _____ and _____ or _____ _____ _____
    added to infant formulas as sweeteners.

24. Diagnosis of botulism is based on:

25. With spinal cord injury, the higher the injury on the spine, the more extensive the damage. Two terms used
    to describe such damage are *paraplegia* and *quadriplegia*. Define these terms.

    a. Paraplegia

    b. Quadriplegia

26. Nursing management of spinal cord injury is concerned with:

    a.

    b.

    c.

27. Treatment with _____ _____ _____ (_____) has
    allowed children greater mobility and functional use of paralyzed muscles to sit, stand, and walk with aid.

APPLYING CRITICAL THINKING TO NURSING PRACTICE

A. Spend a day in a clinic that treats children with cerebral palsy.

    1. What specific nursing goals would help the child with cerebral palsy and the parents?

       a.

       b.

       c.

       d.

       e.

       f.

       g.

2. The child with cerebral palsy has difficulty performing the activities of daily living. Identify the patient goal (a) and the expected outcome (b) related to this problem.

   a.

   b.

3. What is the rationale for the intervention "Demonstrate acceptance of child through own behavior" in relation to body image?

4. What patient goals would address the nursing diagnosis of "Fatique related to increased energy expenditure"?

   a.

   b.

B. Adam, a newborn, is transferred to the pediatric unit for surgical evaluation of a myelomeningocele.

   1. Identify three nursing goals for Adam's initial care.

      a.

      b.

      c.

   2. What evaluative data would indicate the accomplishment of each of the nursing goals identified in question 1?

      a.

      b.

      c.

   3. Because infants with myelomeningocele are at high risk for latex allergy, the nurse would institute "latex precautions." List the behaviors necessary to comply with "latex precautions."

      a.

      b.

C. Spend a day in a clinic serving children with muscular dystrophy.

   1. Because parents of children with muscular dystrophy tend to overprotect their child, how would you intervene to assist both child and family?

2. Because of the genetic etiology of this disease, you would intervene by:

D.   Victor, age 13 years, has been admitted to the pediatric unit with a diagnosis of Guillain-Barrè syndrome.

1. The primary nursing goal is:

2. List at least two nursing interventions to achieve the nursing goal above.

a.

b.

E.   Antonio, age 15 years, is hospitalized in a rehabilitation center for treatment of paraplegia caused by a spinal cord injury.

1. It is important for the nurse to perform a complete assessment to evaluate the extent of the neurologic damage in order to establish a:

2. The nursing goal of rehabilitation for Antonio includes:

Answers

Chapter 1

Review of Essential Concepts

1. a state of complete physical, mental, and social well-being and not merely the absence of disease.
2. a. increase the quality and length of healthy life
   b. eliminate health disparities
3. the number of deaths per 1000 live births during the first year of life
4. last
5. Hong Kong
6. low birth weight
7. unintentional injuries or "accidents"
8. b
9. b
10. new morbidity
11. Abraham Jacobi
12. Lillian Wald
13. Spitz, Robertson
14. a. 2
    b. 4
    c. 3
    d. 6
    e. 1
    f. 5
15. a
16. coordinate, control, multidisciplinary
17. clinical practice guidelines
18. a. therapeutic relationship
    b. family advocacy/caring
    c. disease prevention/health promotion
    d. health teaching
    e. support/counseling
    f. restorative role
    g. coordination/collaboration
    h. ethical decision making
    i. research
    j. health care planning
19. prevention, health teaching
20. purposeful, goal-directed thinking that assists individuals to make judgements based on evidence rather than guesswork
21. a method of problem identification and problem solving that describes what the nurse actually does.
22. a. assessment
    b. nursing diagnosis
    c. planning; outcome identification
    d. implementation
    e. evaluation
23. foundation, decision making

273

24. nursing diagnoses
25. problem statement; etiology; signs, symptoms
26. a. 1
    b. 3
    c. 2
27. dependent, interdependent, independent
28. outcomes, goals
29. a. plans that are sufficiently broad to account for situations that may develop in patients with particular problems
    b. plans that are concerned with only those diagnoses that apply to the particular patient situation
30. implementation
31. evaluation; goal

Applying Critical Thinking to Nursing Practice

A.
1. a. Ensure families' awareness of various health services; inform families of treatments and procedures; involve families in child's care; change or support existing health care practices.
   b. Practice within the overall framework for preventive health; employ an approach of education and anticipatory guidance.
   c. Provide continual assessment and evaluation of the physical status and the emotional and developmental status of the child.
   d. Work with professionals in other disciplines to formulate and implement a plan of care that meets the child's needs.
   e. Determine the least harmful action within the framework of societal mores, professional practice standards, the law, institutional rules, religious traditions, the family's value system, and the nurse's personal values.
   f. Conduct research to provide theoretical foundations for nursing practice and to evaluate the nursing process.

B.
1. Violated: Recognition that the family is the constant in a child's life. The needs of the family members—not just the child—are considered.
2. Violated: Family members and especially siblings should have free access to their family member.
3. Applied: Enabling family members to display their ability and competence. This example fosters a parent-professional partnership.
4. Applied: Empowering the family member to maintain a sense of control over their family's lives.

C.
1. individualized
2. standardized
3. individualized
4. individualized
5. standardized

Chapter 2

Review of Essential Concepts

1. a system that includes children and families, the physical environment, educational facilities, safety and transportation resources, political and governmental agencies, health and social services, communication resources, economic resources, and recreational facilities. The community is also the client of the community health nurse.
2. target populations
3. focusing on promoting and maintaining the health of individuals, families, and groups in the community setting. Community health nursing is a synthesis of nursing and public health. It collaborates with other disciplines to assess, plan, and implement care that emphasizes personal responsibility for health and self-care by community members.
4. population, race/ethnicity, socioeconomic status
5. an increased probability of developing a disease, injury, or illness
6. the science of population health applied to the detection of morbidity and mortality in a population
7. incidence and prevalence
8. Incidence; Prevalence
9. agent, host, environment
10. a. 1
    b. 3
    c. 2
11. benefits
12. objective information
13. community
14. subjective, objective
15. community systems
16. community health diagnosis
17. plan
18. health programs
19. goals, program objectives

Applying Critical Thinking to Nursing Practice

A.
1. primary prevention
2. primary prevention
3. tertiary prevention
4. tertiary prevention
5. secondary prevention
6. secondary prevention

B.
1. health and social services, communication, recreation, physical environment, education, safety and transportation, politics and government, and economics
2. Distribute questionnaires to a sample of people living in the community.
   Interview a sample of community members directly or by telephone.
   Interview community leaders.
3. Conduct a windshield tour. Access records at the chamber of commerce, census bureau, libraries, state health department, Internet sites of voluntary health organizations or government agencies.
4. Decreased immunization levels related to knowledge deficit and barriers to access
5. Within 2 years immunization levels of children under 2 years will be 70%.
6. Structure: Where and by whom is the care delivered in a program?
   Process: Was the care delivered using the operational standards and within the financial guidelines of the program?
   Outcomes: What was the impact to health status? Was there an improvement?

Chapter 3

Review of Essential Concepts

1. whatever the client considers it to be
2. a. Family System Theory: The family is viewed as a system that continually interacts with its members and the environment. The emphasis is on interaction.
   b. Family Stress Theory: This theory explains how families react to stressful events and suggests factors that promote adaptation to stress.
   c. Developmental Theory: This theory uses a family life-cycle approach to compare the changing structure, function, and roles of the family at various stages of development, focusing on time as the central dimension. The theory delineates developmental tasks for the family, much like the individual developmental tasks discussed in relation to personality development.
3. a. 4
   b. 2
   c. 5
   d. 1
   e. 3
4. socialization
5. a. family size
   b. spacing of children
   c. ordinal position in family
   d. multiple births
6. a. true
   b. false
   c. true
7. a. false
   b. true
   c. false
   d. true
8. a. to promote the physical survival and health of the children
   b. to foster the skills and abilities necessary to be a self-sustaining adult
   c. to foster behavioral capabilities for maximizing cultural values and beliefs
9. a. parental age
   b. the quality of the parental relationship
   c. the amount of previous experience with child rearing
   d. parental support systems
   e. effects of stress on parental behavior
10. a. Parents try to control their children's behavior and attitudes through rigid rules and regulations.
    b. Parents allow children to regulate their own activity, viewing themselves as resources for the children, not role models.
    c. Parents combine some practices from both the authoritarian and permissive styles, directing children's behavior and attitudes by emphasizing the reason for rules and negatively reinforcing deviations. Control is focused on the issue. "Inner-directedness" is fostered.
11. a. reasoning
    b. scolding
    c. behavior modification
    d. ignoring
    e. consequences
    f. time-out
    g. corporal punishment
12. a. 3
    b. 6
    c. 1
    d. 5

e. 2

f. 4

13. a. parent-infant attachment

b. the task of telling the child that he or she is adopted

c. the possibility that children may use their adoption as a tool to defy parental authority or as justification for aberrant behavior

14. a. age and sex of the children

b. the outcome of the divorce

c. quality of the parent-child relationship

d. parental care during the years following the divorce

15. true

16. guaranteed time away from work without pay and without jeopardizing their employment to care for their children or parents or spouse in certain situations.

Applying Critical Thinking to Nursing Practice

A.

1. a. Tasks include integrating infants into the family unit, accommodating to new parenting and grandparenting roles, and maintaining the marital bond.

b. Adolescents develop increasing autonomy. Parents refocus on midlife marital and career issues. Parents begin a shift toward concern for the older generation.

2. parental age, father involvement, parenting education

B.

1. events such as marriage, divorce, birth, death, abandonment, and incarceration

2. Roles must be redefined or redistributed.

3. a. commitment

b. appreciation

c. time

d. purpose

e. congruence

f. communication

g. family rules, values, beliefs

h. coping strategies

i. problem solving

j. positive attitude

k. flexibility and adaptability

l. balance

C.

1. Parent may feel guilty about time spent away from children. Parent may feel overburdened by responsibility and demands on time. Parent may feel depressed and doubt ability to cope with emotional needs of child.

2. a. age and sex of child

b. outcome of the divorce

c. quality of the parent-child relationship

d. parental care during years following the divorce

D.

1. Role definitions are altered. Overload is a common source of stress. Time demands and scheduling are major problems.

Chapter 4

Review of Essential Concepts

1. a. 2
   b. 4
   c. 3
   d. 1
2. a. intimate, continued, face-to-face contact; mutual support of the members; and the ability to order or constrain a considerable proportion of individual members' behavior
   b. groups that have limited, intermittent contact and in which there is generally less concern for members' behavior
3. the classification of or affiliation with any of the basic groups or divisions of mankind or any heterogeneous population differentiated by customs, characteristics, language, or similar distinguishing factors
4. ethnocentrism
5. lack of money or material resources, which includes insufficient clothing, poor sanitation, and deteriorating housing
6. social and cultural deprivation, such as limited employment opportunities, inferior educational opportunities, lack of (or inferior) medical services and health care facilities, and an absence of public services
7. 15
8. adolescent
9. Migrant
10. schools
11. a. support
    b. empowerment
    c. boundaries and expectations
    d. constructive use of time
12. a. teaches the child how to deal with dominance and hostility
    b. teaches the children to relate with persons in positions of leadership and authority
    c. relieves the child's boredom
    d. provides recognition that individual members do not receive from teachers and other authority figures
13. the "straddling" of two cultures, which involves the ability to efficiently bridge the gap between an individual culture of origin and the dominant culture
14. geographic, economic
15. feelings of helplessness and discomfort and a state of disorientation experienced by an outsider attempting to comprehend or effectively adapt to a different cultural group because of differences in cultural practices, values, and beliefs
16. a. 4
    b. 1
    c. 3
    d. 2
17. socioeconomic
18. Cultural relativity
19. a. attitude toward time and waiting
    b. person responsible for health care
    c. manner of approach to child
    d. family involvement
    e. tension with members of majority group
    f. verbal and nonverbal communication
    g. level of comfort with body space or distance from others
    h. eye contact
    i. ability to question
    j. terms of address
    k. expression of emotion
    l. food customs

    m. health beliefs

    n. health practices

20. a. 3

    b. 4

    c. 5

    d. 2

    e. 1

21. a. Christian Science

    b. Jehovah's Witness

    c. Roman Catholic

22. a. 3

    b. 2

    c. 4

    d. 1

Applying Critical Thinking to Nursing Practice

A.

1. a. ethnicity

    b. socioeconomic class

    c. religion

    d. schools

    e. communities

    f. peer influences

    g. biculture

2. a. results in a future orientation with the possibility of upward social mobility

    b. results in less reliance on tradition and extended family

    c. results in the child's exposure to a number of adults who differ from one another but who all provide input as role models and teachers

B.

1. a. Hereditary factors may be the result of an inherent lack of resistance to a disease organism (a trait that is an advantage in one environment but places the possessor at a disadvantage in another) or the consequence of intermarriage in a relatively narrow range of geographic, ethnic, or religious restrictions.

    b. Socioeconomic factors include such aspects of impoverished living conditions as crowding, poor sanitation, access to lead-containing substances, and inadequate access to health services.

2. a. results in diet lacking in protein, vitamins, and iron, leading to nutritional deficiency disorders and growth retardation in children

    b. results in family seeking medical care for only serious or life-threatening illness (hence, a lack of preventive health care, dental care, prenatal care, and immunizations)

    c. facilitates transfer of disease

3. Nurses are products of their own cultural backgrounds, which influence their values, thoughts, and actions. When they are aware of their own culturally founded behavior, they are likely to be more sensitive to cultural behavior in others. They tend to identify behaviors as characteristic of a culture rather than as "abnormal" and thus can relate more effectively with the families.

4. a. beliefs about diet and food practices

    b. beliefs regarding birth, death, or other rituals

    c. beliefs regarding medical care

C.

1. orientation to time—some cultures are late for appointments and consider this to be OK

2. person responsible for care—may be mother, father, grandmother, etc.

3. approach to child inappropriate for culture

4. involvement of whole family in visit

5. communication difficulties due to:

language differences

interpretation of eye contact utilized by different cultures

6. health beliefs and practices (such as herbal medicine, coining, etc.) that interfere with assessment and treatment

Chapter 5

Review of Essential Concepts

1. a. 3
   b. 1
   c. 2
   d. 4
2. developmental task
3. a. conception to birth
   b. birth to 28 days
   c. 1 month to 12 months
   d. 1 to 3 years
   e. 3 to 6 years
   f. 6 to 12 years
   g. 10 to 13 years
   h. 13 to 18 years
4. a. cephalocaudal, or head-to-tail
   b. proximodistal, or near-to-far
   c. differentiation, simple to complex
5. sensitive periods
6. predictable
7. false
8. a. 2
   b. 1
   c. 4
   d. 3
9. Double
10. doubles; triples; quadruples
11. sixth
12. false
13. 108, 40, 45
14. a. the difficult child
    b. the slow-to-warm-up child
    c. the easy child
15. a. 2
    b. 1
    c. 3
    d. 4
    e. 5
16. a. trust vs. mistrust
    b. autonomy vs. shame and doubt
    c. initiative vs. guilt
    d. industry vs. inferiority
    e. identity vs. identity confusion
17. a. 3, 5
    b. 1, 8
    c. 4, 7
    d. 2, 6
18. comprehension, expressed

19. a. preconventional morality
    b. postconventional level
    c. conventional level
20. includes all the notions, beliefs, and convictions that constitute an individual's self-knowledge and that influence the individual's relationships with others
21. body image
22. self-esteem
23. a. 2
    b. 5
    c. 1
    d. 4
    e. 3
24. a. sensorimotor development
    b. intellectual development
    c. socialization
    d. creativity
    e. self-awareness
    f. therapeutic value
    g. moral value
25. true
26. developmental delays
27. socioeconomic level
28. "an imbalance between environmental demands and a person's coping resources that . . . disrupts the equilibrium of the person."
29. Television
30. a. You are smarter than what you see on your television.
    b. Television world is not real.
    c. Television teaches that some people are more important than others.
    d. Television keeps doing the same things over and over again.
    e. Somebody is always trying to make money with televsion.
31. knowledgeable

Applying Critical Thinking to Nursing Practice

A.
1. No. It should quadruple to 28 lbs.
2. Yes. His current height is 50% of eventual adult height.
3. yes; yes

B.
1. Although children vary in both their rate of growth and their acquisition of developmental skills, certain predictable patterns are universal and basic to all human beings.
2. a. trust vs. mistrust (consistently meet the child's basic needs; provide loving care)
   b. autonomy vs. shame and doubt (allow the child the opportunity to make choices)
   c. initiative vs. guilt (encourage exploration of the environment; set realistic limits)
   d. industry vs. inferiority (encourage competition and cooperation; assist in setting achievable goals)
   e. identity vs. role confusion (provide positive feedback regarding appearance and activities)
3. a. no concept of right or wrong evident
   b. imitation of religious gestures and behaviors of others without comprehension of meaning
   c. imitation of religious behavior and following of parental religious beliefs as part of daily lives without real understanding of basic concepts
   d. strong interest in religion with acceptance of a deity; petitions to this deity made and expected to be answered
   e. realization that prayers are not always answered; initiation of modification or abandonment of religious practices; questioning of the religious standards of their parents

C.

1. Infants with difficult or slow-to-warm-up patterns of behavior are more vulnerable to the development of behavioral problems in early and middle childhood. However, any child can develop behavioral problems if there is dissonance between his or her temperament and the environment. When parents are unable to accept and deal with the child's behavior, there is a greater likelihood of subsequent behavioral problems.

2. a. even-tempered, regular, and predictable habits; positive approach to new stimuli; adaptability to change
   b. highly active; irritable; irregular in habits; has negative withdrawal responses; slow to adapt to new routines, people, or situations

D.

1. a. Provide a positive role model by developing television substitutes such as reading, athletics, physical conditioning, and hobbies.
   b. Construct a time chart of the child's activities.
   c. Discuss with the child what both believe to be a balanced set of activities.
   d. At the beginning of each week, select appropriate programs from television schedules.
   e. Allow the child to select programs from this approved list.
   f. Limit the child's viewing to 2 hours or less per day.
   g. Rule out TV at specific times.
   h. Make a list of alternate activities.
   i. Require that the child choose to do something from this list before watching television.
   j. Watch programs with the child.
   k. Discuss program and commercial content with the child.
   l. Distiquish between the real and unreal.
   m. Correlate consequences with actions.
   n. Point out subtle messages.
   o. Explore alternatives to aggressive conflict resolution.
   p. Stress the purpose of the program.
   q. Explain likes and dislikes.
   r. Turn the TV off after the selected program is over.
   s. Monitor cable and pay TV selections.
   t. Limit use of TV as a safe distraction to potentially stressful times.

Chapter 6

Review of Essential Concepts

1. a. Verbal communication involves language and its expression, as well as vocalizations in the form of laughs, moans, or squalls.
   b. Nonverbal communication is often called "body language" and includes gestures, movements, facial expressions, postures, and reactions.
   c. Abstract communication takes the form of play, artistic expression, symbols, photographs, and choice of clothing.
2. private; minimum distractions; play opportunities for children while parent is interviewed
3. Triage
4. a. allows the nurse to obtain information concerning the health and developmental status of the child, factors that may influence the child's life, and cues to aspects in the child's health and development that may be a source of concern to the parents
   b. permits the nurse to allow for maximum freedom of expression while not allowing the interview to go off on tangents
   c. allows the nurse to make objective judgments concerning the perception of the parents, is useful in preventing the nurse's views from being interjected into the interview process, and aids in detecting cues from the parents that may aid in identifying problem areas
   d. allows the interviewee to sort out thoughts and feelings
   e. allows the nurse to see the problem from the parents' perspective

    f. facilitates the formulation of solutions, because in order for a problem to be solved, the nurse and parent must agree that one exists

    g. includes the parents in the problem-solving process and allows solutions to be proposed that will be adhered to by parents

    h. provides preventive methods so that problems will not occur

    i. allows the nurse to recognize and prevent blocks that may alter the quality of the helping relationship

5. Learn proper terms of address.

   Use a positive tone of voice to convey interest.

   Speak slowly and carefully, not loudly.

   Encourage questions.

   Learn basic words and sentences of the family's language.

   Avoid professional jargon.

   Explain the reason for questions and how information will be used.

   Repeat important information more than once.

   Always give reason or purpose for a treatment.

   Use information written in the family's language.

   Offer the services of an interpreter.

   Learn methods of communicating from families and representatives of their culture.

   Address intergenerational needs.

   Be sincere, open, and honest.

6. Any three of the following are acceptable answers:

   Long periods of silence

   Wide eyes and fixed facial expression

   Constant fidgeting or attempting to move away

   Nervous habits (e.g., tapping)

   Sudden disruptions

   Looking around

   Yawning

   Frequently looking at a watch or clock

   Attempting to change topic of discussion

7. cultural, legal, ethical

8. a. true

    b. false

    c. true

    d. true

9. a. 2

    b. 1

    c. 3

    d. 4

10. a. Spend time together.

    b. Encourage expression of ideas and feelings.

    c. Respect their views.

    d. Tolerate differences.

    e. Praise good points.

    f. Respect their privacy.

    g. Set a good example.

11. d

12. writing, drawing, magic, play

13. a. identifying information

    b. chief complaint (CC)

    c. present illness (PI)

    d. past history (PH)

    e. review of systems (ROS)

    f. family medical history

    g. psychosocial history

    h. sexual history

    i. family history

    j. nutritional assessment

14. a. approximate weight at 6 months, 1 year, 2 years, and 5 years of age
    b. approximate length at ages 1 and 4 years
    c. dentition, including age of onset, number of teeth, and symptoms during teething
    d. developmental milestones
15. a. family composition
    b. home and community environment
    c. occupation and education of family members
    d. cultural and religious traditions
16. sociogram
17. a. family interactions and roles
    b. power, decision making, and problem solving
    c. communication
    d. expression of feelings and individuality
18. adaptation, partnership, growth, affection, resolve (commitment)
19. dietary intake, clinical examination
20. c

Applying Critical Thinking to Nursing Practice

A.

1. The first component to this process is an introduction of the interviewer to the parents.
2. It is important to include the parent in the problem-solving process because a parent who is included will be more likely to follow through on a course of action.
3. Some of the more common blocks to communication are socializing, giving unrestricted advice, offering inappropriate reassurance, giving overready encouragement defending a situation or opinion, using stereotypic comments, using close-ended questions, interrupting the client, talking more than the interviewee, forming prejudged conclusions, and deliberately changing the focus.
4. A number of techniques are effective. These include "I" messages; third-person technique; facilitative responding; storytelling; using books, dreams, "what if" questions, three wishes, rating games, word association games, sentence completion, pros and cons; and writing, drawing, magic, and play.

B.

1. Learn proper terms of address.
   Use a positive tone of voice to convey interest.
   Speak slowly and carefully, not loudly.
   Encourage questions.
   Learn basic words and sentences of the family's language.
   Avoid professional terms.
   Explain why questions are being asked.
   Repeat important information more than once.
   Always give reason or purpose for a treatment.
   Use information written in the family's language.
   Offer the services of an interpreter when necessary.
   Learn from families and representatives of their culture various methods of communicating information.
   Address intergenerational needs.
   Be sincere, open, and honest.
2. The nurse can redirect the focus of the interview by saying that they can talk about the other children later in the interview.
3. Since Susan has been in this country only 6 months, she may not have received her immunizations. It is extremely important for the nurse to obtain an accurate record of immunizations from Mrs. Fernandez.
4. The nurse should obtain information concerning the age, marital status, state of health, presence of illness, cause of death if deceased, and any evidence of heart disease, etc., of first-degree relatives.

5. a. HOME (home observation for management of the environment)
   b. HSQ (Home Screening Questionnaire)
C.
   1. The three methods include 24-hour recall, food diary, and food frequency record.
   2. Anthropometry is the measurement of height, weight, head circumference, proportions, skinfold thickness, and arm circumference. Skinfold thickness is a measurement of the body's fat content and would be useful in determining whether Gwen is obese.
   3. a. altered nutrition: more than body requirements related to eating practices
      b. altered nutrition: more than body requirements related to knowledge deficit of parents

Chapter 7

Review of Essential Concepts

1. a. minimizing the stress and anxiety associated with body part assessment
   b. fostering a trusting nurse-child-parent relationship
   c. allowing for maximum preparation of the child
   d. preserving the essential security of the parent-child relationship
   e. maximizing the accuracy and reliability of the assessment findings
2. a. Assess the child for reasons for uncooperative behavior.
   b. Try to involve the child and parent in the process.
   c. Avoid prolonged explanations about the examining procedure.
   d. Use a firm, direct approach regarding expected behavior.
   e. Perform the examination as quickly as possible.
   f. Have an attendant gently restrain the child.
   g. Minimize any disruptions or stimulation.
   h. Limit the number of people in the room.
   i. Use an isolated room.
   j. Use a quiet, calm, confident voice.
3. a. growth measurements
   b. physiologic measurements
   c. general appearance
   d. skin
   e. lymph nodes
   f. head and neck
   g. eyes
   h. ears
   i. nose
   j. mouth and throat
   k. chest
   l. lungs
   m. heart
   n. abdomen
   o. genitalia
   p. anus
   q. back and extremities
   r. neurologic assessment
   s. developmental assessment
4. d
5. respiration, pulse, temperature
6. for a full minute
7. apically

8. a. 2
   b. 3
   c. 4
   d. 1
9. When assessing the head of an 8-month-old, the nurse should record the general shape, symmetry, head control, head posture, motion, presence of patent sutures, fontanels, fractures, swelling, and symmetry and movement of the face.
10. a. 3
    b. 1
    c. 2
    d. 4
11. b
12. translucent, light pearly pink or gray
13. false
14. a. vesicular
    b. bronchovesicular
    c. bronchial
15. crackles, wheezes
16. point of maximum intensity
17. peristalsis, bowel sounds
18. hair
19. lateral curvature of the spine
20. false
21. a. 2
    b. 3
    c. 1
    d. 4
22. true
23. false

Applying Critical Thinking to Nursing Practice

A.
1. You should observe Tia for signs of readiness such as her willingness to talk to you, make eye contact, accept the offered equipment, allow physical contact, or choose to sit on the examining table. Several methods might be used to facilitate the exam process. You could tell a story or use a puppet. Since Tia needs to have a developmental assessment, you might want to begin with this aspect of the exam because it might be perceived by Tia as a game.
2. Tia is 3 years of age, so she can have her height taken while standing. She should be encouraged to stand as tall and straight as possible.
3. Additional assessment information might include Tia's parents' patterns of growth, whether her growth pattern has been steady, and her nutritional intake.
4. Tia may not understand that she should not bite down on the thermometer or that she has to keep the thermometer under her tongue and her mouth closed.
5. Tia should have a complete vision assessment that includes binocularity and acuity. To test for binocularity, you might use the corneal light reflex test or the cover test. To test for acuity, you might use the Tumbling E test or the Allen cards.

B.
1. After the general appearance section, the skin is assessed.
2. The infant's height is obtained in the recumbent position by fully extending the child's body. The school-age child's height is obtained by having the child stand straight. Height should be recorded to the nearest 1/8 in. or 1 mm.
3. Radial pulses can be obtained if the child is over 2 years of age. The infant's pulse should be taken apically, and the school-age child's can be taken radially.
4. Information in this area includes the child's personality; level of activity; reaction to stress, requests, frustration; interaction with others; degree of alertness; and response to stimuli.

5. Hearing ability should be assessed.
6. quality, intensity, rate, rhythm
7. Instruct the child to hold his or her breath. In sinus arrhythmia this causes the heart rate to remain steady.

C.
1. The parent is told that the purpose of the test is to help the nurse observe what the child can do at this age and that the results of the performance will be explained after all items have been completed. It should be emphasized that this is not an intelligence test.
2. The parent is asked whether the child's performance is typical of his or her behavior at other times.
3. A delay is determined by failure on an item completely to the left of the age line.
4. Items are scored as follows: P, passing; F, failing; and R, refusal.
5. All children with questionable or abnormal results should be rescreened before a referral for further diagnostic testing is made.

Chapter 8

Review of Essential Concepts

1. the entrance of air into the upper airway, replacing the lung fluid, and initiation of breathing.
2. false
3. a
4. a. large surface area
   b. thin layer of subcutaneous fat
   c. inability to shiver
5. seven; twice
6. d
7. true
8. a. skin and mucous membranes
   b. cellular elements of immunologic system
   c. antibodies
9. a. heart rate
   b. respiratory effort
   c. muscle tone
   d. reflex irritability
   e. color
10. 10
11. birth weight, gestational age
12. false
13. true
14. posture, behavior, skin, head, eyes, ears, nose, mouth and throat, neck, chest, lungs, heart, abdomen, genitalia, back and anus, extremities, and neurologic system
15. b
16. 6, 8
17. an alert and active infant, increased heart and respiratory rate, active gag reflex, increased gastric and respiratory secretions, and passage of meconium
18. Brazelton Neonatal Behavioral Assessment Scale (BNBAS)
19. true
20. a. maintenance of patent airway
    b. maintenance of stable body temperature
    c. protection from injury and infection
    d. provision of optimum nutrition
    e. promotion of parent-infant attachment
    f. preparation for discharge and home care

21. true
22. Soap alters the pH of the skin surface, which is slightly acidic, and alters "acid mantle."
23. false
24. b
25. Human milk
26. true
27. Postpartum hospitalizations are shorter.

Applying Critical Thinking to Nursing Practice

A.
  1. heart rate, respiratory effort, muscle tone, reflex irritability, and color
  2. below 100 beats/min
  3. 7, 10
  4. The behaviors that are observed include an initial period of alertness, vigorous suck, initially elevated heart and respiratory rates, active bowel sounds, and falling temperature.
  5. c
B.
  1. Perinatal mortality and morbidity are related to gestational age and weight.
  2. posture, square window, arm recoil, popliteal angle, scarf sign, and heel-to-ear maneuver
  3. his or her weight falls between the 10th and 90th percentile
C.
  1. 33 and 35 cm (13 to 14 inches); microcephaly or craniostenosis should be suspected
  2. The areas to assess include symmetry of the eyes, presence of tears, presence of discharge, presence of corneal reflex, presence of pupillary reflex, presence of nystagmus or strabismus, color of the iris, and presence of edema in the eyelids.
  3. The infant's eyes are closed, and the infant has irregular breathing, has slight muscular twitching of the body, has rapid eye movements under closed eyelids, and may smile.
D.
  1. Any three of the following diagnoses are acceptable:
     Ineffective airway clearance related to excess mucus, improper positioning
     Risk for altered body temperature related to immature temperature control, change in environmental temperature
     Risk for infection related to deficient immunologic defenses, environmental factors, maternal disease
     Risk for trauma related to physical helplessness
     Altered nutrition, less than body requirements (potential), related to immaturity, parental knowledge deficit
     Altered family processes related to maturational crisis, birth of term infant, change in family unit
  2. Any four of the following interventions are acceptable:
     Suction the mouth and nasopharynx with bulb syringe.
     Position the infant on his or her right side after feeding.
     Position the infant on his or her back during sleep.
     Perform as few procedures as possible on the infant during the first hour of life.
     Take vital signs.
     Observe for signs of respiratory distress.
     Keep diapers, clothing, and blankets loose.
     Clean nares of crusted material.
     Check for patency of nares.
  3. The reason that clothes are kept loose is that infants are abdominal breathers; this intervention allows for maximal expansion of the lungs and avoids overheating.
  4. Criteria includes: airway remains patent, breathing that is regular and unlabored, normal respiratory rate.
  5. The parents should be instructed in routine baby care such as feeding, bathing, and umbilical and circumcision care. They should also be encouraged to participate in parenting classes, and the use of car restraints should be discussed.

E.
1. Specific behaviors that might be assessed include the following: the parent reaching out for the baby when she is brought into the room, referring to the infant by name, talking about who the child looks like, speaking about the uniqueness of the infant, the type of body contact used, types of stimulation, and whether or not the parents avoid eye contact.
2. altered family processes related to maturational crisis, birth of term infant, change in family unit
3. Any six of the following interventions are acceptable:
   Allow parents to see and hold the infant as soon as possible.
   Perform eye care after the parents have met the infant.
   Identify the infant's unique behaviors.
   Encourage parents to "talk out" their labor and delivery experience.
   Identify behavioral steps in the attachment process.
   Encourage the family to room in.
   Observe and assess the reciprocity of cues between the infant and parents.
   Assist parents in recognizing attention-nonattention cycles.
   Assess variables affecting the attachment process.

Chapter 9

Review of Essential Concepts

1. presenting part, maternal pelvis
2. a
3. the clavicle or collar bone
4. facial nerve paralysis—pressure on the facial nerve, cranial nerve VII during delivery, causing facial nerve paralysis
5. proper positioning of the affected arm
6. a. true
   b. true
   c. true
   d. false
7. a. 4
   b. 3
   c. 2
   d. 1
8. a. birth weight (size)
   b. gestational age
   c. mortality (predominant pathophysiologic problems)
9. Determine presence of abdominal distention or visible peristalsis.
   Determine any signs of regurgitation and time related to feeding.
   Describe amount, color, consistency, and odor of any emesis.
   Palpate liver margin.
   Describe amount, color, consistency of stools.
   Describe bowel sounds (presence or absence).
10. weighing
11. cold stress
12. higher
13. size, condition
14. energy
15. acid mantle of the skin
16. a. tactile
    b. auditory
    c. vestibular

    d. olfactory

    e. gustatory

    f. visual

17. physiologic changes, behavioral observations
18. Neonatal Pain, Agitation, and Sedation Scale
19. parent the infant in any way they wish to (touch, hold, talk to, etc.)
20. a. 1
    b. 3
    c. 2
21. jaundice or icterus
22. This occurs because of the immaturity of hepatic function combined with increased hemolysis of excess red blood cells.
23. phototherapy
24. Rh, ABO
25. prevention, Rho-immune globulin (RhIg) (Rhogam)
26. c
27. congenital heart
28. a. metabolic disorder
    b. toxic disturbances
    c. prenatal infections
    d. postnatal infections
    e. trauma at birth
    f. congenital malformations
    g. miscellaneous disorders
29. true
30. intestinal ischemia, colonization by pathogenic bacteria, and substrate in intestine
31. abdominal distention, blood in stools or gastric contents, gastric retention, localized abdominal wall erythema or induration, bilious vomitus
32. d
33. phenobarbital, chlorpromazine, clonidine, diazepam, methadone, and morphine
34. Toxoplasmosis, Other, Rubella, Cytomegalovirus infection, Herpes simplex, Syphilis
35. syndrome
36. alcohol, tobacco, antiepileptics, isotretinoin, lithium, cocaine, and diethylstibesterol
37. IEMs
38. true
39. phenylalanine hydroxylase
40. screening with the Guthrie blood test
41. false

Applying Critical Thinking to Nursing Practice

A.

  1. a. A vaguely outlined area of edematous tissue situated over the portion of the scalp that presents in a vertex delivery. The swelling consists of serum, blood, or both, accumulated in the tissues above the bone, and it may extend beyond the bone margins. It is present within 24 hours of birth.

    b. Formed when blood vessels rupture during labor or delivery to produce bleeding into the area between the bone and its periosteum. The boundaries are sharply demarcated and do not extend beyond the limits of the bone. Swelling is usually minimal at birth and increases on the second or third day.

  2. a. detection of complications

    b. parental support

B.

  1. The most meaningful method of classification is one that encompasses all three methods (i.e., birth weight, gestational age, pathophysiologic problems).

  2. High-risk infants have deficient immunologic defenses and are also exposed to many sources of nosocomial infections.

3. altered nutrition (less than body requirements) related to inability to ingest nutrients because of immaturity and/or illness
4. The infant should be weighed daily and should exhibit a steady weight gain.
5. Assessment of the skin reveals that the skin remains clean and intact with no evidence of irritation or injury.
6. a. keeping parents informed of infant's progress
   b. facilitating parent-infant attachment
   c. facilitating sibling-infant attachment
   d. prepare for home care
7. Since the infant is in an ICU, the parents may not have had time to become acquainted with and attached to their infant. Encouraging visitation counteracts interruptions of the bonding process and keeps parents informed of the infant's progress.

C.
1. a. immaturity of hepatic function
   b. increased bilirubin load from increased hemolysis of red blood cells
2. a. after 24 hours
   b. by the third day
   c. by the fifth day
3. a. Shield the infant's eyes with an opaque mask.
   b. Place the infant nude under the fluorescent light with a plexiglas shield.
   c. Monitor body temperature.
   d. Give additional fluids.
   e. Provide meticulous skin care.

D.
1. Through cross-contamination. The sources of this could include humidifying apparatus, suction machines, indwelling catheters, poor handwashing.
2. Some of the signs of sepsis are poor temperature control, pallor, hypotension, edema, respiratory distress, diminished or increased activity, full fontanel, poor feeding, vomiting, diarrhea, jaundice, and an infant not doing well.
3. recognition of the existing problem

E.
1. Michael was premature and experienced intestinal ischemia.
2. early recognition
3. lethargy, poor feeding, hypotension, vomiting, apnea, decreased urinary output, unstable temperature, and jaundice

F.
1. It occurs as a result of the hyperplasia and hypertrophy of the islet cells in utero. The islet cells continue to excrete large amounts of insulin after birth, resulting in decreased blood glucose levels (hypoglycemia).
2. Feeding is begun early to prevent hypoglycemia.
3. a. brachial plexus injury and palsy
   b. fractured clavicle
   c. phrenic nerve palsy

Chapter 10

Review of Essential Concepts

1. doubled
2. d
3. a. greater proportion of extracellular fluid
   b. immaturity of renal function
4. 4 months
5. b
6. a
7. true
8. primary, secondary
9. a. the ability to distinguish the mother from other individuals
   b. the achievement of object permanence
10. true
11. preference for mother demonstrated by behaviors such as clinging to the parent, crying, and turning away from the stranger
12. 9, 10
13. psychosocial
14. mirrors, bright toys to hold, rattles or bells, soft squeeze toys, mobiles, and swings
15. false
16. age of child in months minus 6 = number of teeth at this age
17. protection
18. iron
19. false
20. a. The digestive tract is not mature enough.
    b. Food allergies may develop.
    c. The extrusion reflex is still strong.
21. infant cereal; because of its high iron content
22. true
23. a
24. false
25. local tenderness, erythema, and swelling at the injection site; a low-grade fever; and behavioral changes
26. asphyxiation by aspiration of foreign material
27. automobile injuries

Applying Critical Thinking to Nursing Practice

A.
1. Yes. Jerry should have at least doubled his birth weight by at least 5 months of age.
2. Jerry's developmental milestones are assessed as follows: when supine, lifts head off table, sits erect momentarily, bears full weight on feet, transfers objects from hand to hand, rakes at a small object, bangs cube on table, produces vowel sounds and chained syllables, vocalizes four distinct vowel sounds, plays peekaboo, fears strangers when mother disappears, and imitates simple acts.
3. You should stress to Mrs. Backer that this behavior is normal and indicates good parental attachment. Mrs. Backer should be encouraged to allow clingy behavior and to encourage close friends or relatives to visit often.
4. a. frozen teething ring to chew on
   b. topical analgesics such as Baby Ora-Jel
5. Jerry's lack of interest in breast-feeding may indicate his desire to be weaned. You should suggest that Jerry might be weaned to a cup, that it should be done gradually by replacing one feeding at a time, with the nighttime feeding the last to be replaced, and not allowing the child to take a bottle to bed.

6. a. Clean teeth with a damp cloth.
    b. Do not include concentrated sugars in the diet.
    c. Do not coat pacifiers with honey.
    d. Never allow a bottle to be taken to bed or during a nap.

B.
1. associates nipple with parent's voice and stops crying, grasps objects reflexively, showing great interest in mirror image
2. a. the reason for the concern
    b. the frequency and duration of waking
    c. the usual bedtime routine
    d. the number of nighttime feedings
    e. the interventions Rachel's mother attempted
3. a. Rachel should be started on cereal first.
    b. Cereal should be mixed with formula.
    c. Spoon-feeding should be first introduced after the infant has had some formula.
    d. The infant will at first push the spoon away, but be persistent.
    e. Introduce new foods one at a time. New foods are fed in small amounts (about 1 tsp.) and for a period of 4 to 7 days.
    f. As the amount of solids increases, she should decrease the amount of formula.
    g. Do not introduce foods by mixing them with formula in the bottle.

C.
1. a. Ensure proper storage such as refrigeration and protection from exposure to light.
    b. Ensure protection from exposure to light.
2. The safest site for the administration of immunizations is the vastus lateralis or ventrogluteal.

D.
1. Such developmental landmarks include crawling, standing, cruising, walking, climbing, pulling on objects, throwing objects, picking up small objects, exploring by mouthing, exploring away from parent.
2. a. Place guard around heating appliances, fireplace, or furnace.
    b. Keep electrical wires hidden.
    c. Place plastic guards over electrical outlets; place furniture in front of outlets.
    d. Keep hanging tablecloth out of reach.
    e. Apply a sunscreen when infant is exposed to sunlight.
3. The infant is now mobile and could drown in a tub if allowed to get in the bathroom.
4. Infants at this age still explore objects by mouthing them and might choke on a small object.
5. The child may think the medication is candy and eat some and might accidentally be poisoned.
6. You should suggest that the grandparents' homes be accident-proofed as well.

Chapter 11

Review of Essential Concepts

1. increased
2. 10 or more times the Recommended Dietary Allowances
3. 0.4 mg folic acid daily
4. b
5. true
6. loss of appetite, diminished taste sensation, delayed healing, skin lesions, alopecia, diarrhea, growth failure, and retarded sexual maturity
7. lacto-ovovegetarian
8. inadequate protein for growth; inadequate calories for energy and growth; poor digestibility; deficiencies of vitamins and minerals
9. Food Guide Pyramid

10. 30
11. a. inadequate food intake
    b. diarrhea
12. d
13 a. food allegy or hypersensenstive—immunologic causes
    b. food intolerance—nonimmunologic causes
14. allergy with heriditary tendency
15. eliminate milk followed by a challenge test after improvement of symptoms
16. lactase
17. abdominal pain, bloating, flatus, diarrhea (severity may range from mild to severe)
18. a. 2
    b. 3
    c. 1
19. a. infant's diet
    b. diet of the breast-feeding mother
    c. time of day when attacks occur
    d. relationship of the attack to feeding times
    e. presence of specific family members during attacks and habits such as smoking by family members
    f. activity of caregiver before, during, and after the crying
    g. characteristics of the cry
    h. measures used to relieve the crying and their effectiveness
    i. the infant's stooling, voiding, and sleep patterns
20. false
21. a. isolation and social crisis
    b. inadequate support system
    c. poor parenting models as a child
22. the provision of adequate nutrition for growth
23. a. Provide a primary core of staff to feed the child.
    b. Provide a quiet, unstimulating environment.
    c. Maintain a calm, even temperament.
    d. Talk to the child by giving directions about eating.
    e. Be persistent.
    f. Maintain a face-to-face posture with the child.
    g. Introduce new foods slowly.
    h. Follow the child's rhythm of feeding.
    i. Develop a structured routine.
24. supine
25. positional plagiocephaly
26. to avoid any suggestions of responsibility on the part of the parents
27. apparent (or acute) life-threatening event
28. cardiopneumogram or pneumocardiogram
29. continuous cardiorespiratory home monitoring
30. a. removal of leads from infant when not attached to monitor
    b. unplugging power cord from electrical outlet when not plugged into monitor
    c. using safety covers on electrical outlets

Applying Critical Thinking to Nursing Practice

A.
  1. The nurse should have assessed the cultural food preferences of the Morrisons. Since they are vegetarians, they may have a lack of knowledge of how to meet their child's nutritional needs on this type of diet.
  2. exactly what the diet includes and excludes

3. a. teaching the Morrisons to include grains, beans, milk products (if allowed) to meet protein and niacin requirements
   b. teaching the Morrisons to include iron-fortified cereals until child is 18 months old
   c. teaching the Morrisons to include juices containing vitamin C
   d. suggesting that they use soy-based formulas
   e. suggesting that they use a variety of foods in the diet
4. If the interventions were successful, the infant would begin to gain weight; the infant would not exhibit signs of niacin deficiency such as scaly dermatitis, diarrhea, or apathy; and the parents would be able to verbalize and provide a nutritionally adequate diet for the child.

B.
1. a. correct nutritional deficit to achieve ideal weight for height
   b. allow for catch-up growth
   c. restore optimum body composition
   d. educate parents regarding the child's nutritional requirements and appropriate feeding methods
2. a. the child achieves ideal weight for height
   b   parents verbalize appropriate nutritional requirements
   c. parents demonstrate appropriate feeding techniques

C.
1. a. Ask parents only factual questions.
   b. Avoid making any remarks that suggest responsibility.
   c. Discuss the need for an autopsy.
   d. Allow parents to say good-bye to their child.
2. a. Make a professional home visit as soon as possible.
   b. Provide literature about SIDS.
   c. Make a referral to other parents who have lost infants.

D.
1. Monitors can cause electrical burns and electrocution.
2. The utility company is informed because if there is a power outage, some provision of emergency power may be provided. The rescue squad is notified because in the event that the infant stops breathing, they will be aware of the problem, and help may arrive more quickly.
3. used, response

Chapter 12

Review of Essential Concepts

1. 12 months, 36 months
2. 2 $1/2$
3. true
4. because the abdominal musculature is not yet well-developed and because the legs, though elongating, are still short in relation to the rest of the body and retain a slightly bowed or curved appearance
5. 20/40
6. elimination
7. development of locomotion
8. a. differentiation of self from others, particularly the mother
   b. toleration of separation from the parent
   c. ability to withstand delayed gratification
   d. control over bodily functions
   e. acquisition of socially acceptable behavior
   f. verbal means of communication
   g. ability to interact with others in a less egocentric manner
9. autonomy, doubt, shame

10. a. negativism
    b. ritualism
11. tolerate delayed gratification
12. e
13. preconceptual phase
14. a
15. a. 2
    b. 3
    c. 1
    d. 5
    e. 4
16. true
17. a. the child's emergence from a symbiotic fusion with the mother
    b. those achievements that mark children's assumption of their own individual characteristics in the environment
18. false
19. 300, 65
20. independence
21. parallel
22. d
23. quadrupled
24. 18, 24
25. true
26. firstborn
27. false
28. include
29. independence
30. the opportunities of a "no" answer
31. physiologic anorexia
32. 1 tablespoon
33. brushing, flossing
34. fluoride, reduced
35. true
36. d
37. Injuries
38. There is a need to emphasize safety awareness in parents.
39. 20, 1
40. 60, 8
41. Scalds
42. improper storage of toxic agents

Applying Critical Thinking to Nursing Practice

A.
1. a. slightly below the 75th percentile
   b. falls at the 75th percentile
2. Growth slows considerably during the toddler years. A toddler gains approximately 4 to 6 pounds and grows 3 inches per year. Growth occurs in spurts and plateaus during toddlerhood.
3. a. goes up and down stairs alone, using both feet on each step; runs fairly well, with a wide stance; picks up objects without falling; and can kick a ball forward without overbalancing
   b. can build a tower of six to seven cubes; aligns two or more cubes like a train; turns the pages of a book one at a time; can imitate vertical and circular strokes when drawing; and turns doorknob and unscrews lid
   c. has vocabulary of 300 words; uses two- to three-word phrases; uses the pronouns I, me, and you; understands directional commands; gives first name; verbalizes need for toileting; and talks incessantly

4. This is characteristic of parallel play, which is typical during the toddler years.
5. a. Toys should be purchased using safety and developmental level as guidelines.
   b. The child should be allowed to choose the toys he wishes to play with at a given time.
6. b
7. a. If drinking water is not fluoridated, provide fluoride supplements.
   b. Arrange a visit to the dentist so that the child may become familiar with the equipment.
   c. Introduce the use of a soft toothbrush as part of the child's bedtime regimen.
   d. Encourage the consumption of a low-cariogenic diet.

B.
1. by their persistent "no" response to every request
2. negative response
3. As an assertion of self-control and an attempt to control the environment, it increases independence.
4. Toddlers assert their independence by violently objecting in this manner to restrictions on their behavior.
5. Because the growth rate slows, there is a decrease in nutritional needs.
6. a. unpredictable table manners
   b. rituals involving mealtime and utensils
   c. inability to sit through family mealtimes
   d. food fads or jags
7. because the eating habits established in the first 2 or 3 years of life tend to have lasting effects
8. fears of separation
9. a. bedtime rituals
   b. use of transitional objects

C.
1. a. child protection
   b. parent education
2. The toddler experiences unrestricted freedom because of increased locomotion and is unaware of danger in the environment.
3. a. motor vehicle injuries
   b. drowning
   c. burns
   d. poisoning
   e. falls
   f. choking and suffocation
   g. bodily damage
4. a. matches and cigarette lighters
   b. sources of water—tubs, swimming pools
   c. medications, toxic agents, plants
   d. unguarded stairways
   e. tools, garden equipment, and firearms
5. a. 4, 7, 9
   b. 1, 4, 5, 6
   c. 3, 8
   d. 2, 4, 5, 7
6. Motor vehicle injuries; approved restraints properly installed and applied can reduce fatalities and injuries.

Chapter 13

Review of Essential Concepts

1. 3, fifth
2. slow, stabilize
3. true
4. initiative
5. superego
6. readiness
7. a. the preconceptual phase (ages 2 to 4 years)
   b. the phase of intuitive thought (ages 4 to 7 years)
8. There is a shift from totally egocentric thought to social awareness and ability to consider other viewpoints.
9. Speech
10. Causality resembles logical thought. Preschoolers explain a concept as they heard it described by others, but their understanding is limited.
11. magical
12. true
13. a. They can relate to unfamiliar people easily.
    b. They tolerate brief separations from parents with little or no protest.
14. true
15. 2100
16. telegraphic
17. a. The preschooler is able to verbalize his or her request for independence.
    b. The preschooler can perform many tasks independently.
18. associative
19. $2\frac{1}{2}$, 3
20. a. They become friends for the child in times of loneliness.
    b. They accomplish what the child is still attempting.
    c. They experience what the child wants to forget or remember.
21. a
22. a. learning group cooperation
    b. adjusting to various sociocultural differences
    c. coping with frustration, dissatisfaction, and anger
23. a. whether the facility is licensed
    b. qualifications of the staff
    c. student-to-staff ratio
    d. discipline policy
    e. environmental safety precautions
    f. provision of meals
    g. sanitary conditions
    h. adequate indoor and outdoor space per child
    i. fee schedule
    j. health practices of agency
24. personal observation
25. a. Determine what the child knows and thinks.
    b. Be honest with responses.
26. Masturbation
27. a. fear of the dark
    b. fear of being left alone
    c. fear of animals
    d. fear of ghosts
    e. fear of sexual matters
    f. fear of objects or persons associated with pain

28. refers to behavior that attempts to hurt a person or destroy property
29. a. quantity (number of occurrences)
    b. severity (interference with function)
    c. distribution (different manifestations)
    d. onset (sudden change in behavior)
    e. duration (at least 4 weeks)
30. 2, 4
31. The child is using his rapidly growing vocabulary faster than he can produce the words. The failure to master sensorimotor integrations results in stuttering or stammering.
32. true
33. true
34. 5
35. Four
36. The quality of the food consumed is more important than the quantity.
37. false
38. a. to preserve the temporary teeth
    b. to teach good dental habits
39. true

Applying Critical Thinking to Nursing Practice

A.
 1. a. slightly above the 25th percentile
    b. falls at the 25th percentile
 2. Physical growth slows and stabilizes during this time. The average weight gain is about 5 lb (2.3 kg) per year, and height increases by about 2.5 to 3 in. (6.75 to 7.5 cm) per year.
 3. a. skips and hops on alternate feet; throws and catches ball well; jumps rope; skates with good balance; walks backward with heel to toe; jumps from height of 12 inches and lands on toes; balances on alternate feet with eyes closed
    b. ties shoelaces; uses scissors well; copies a diamond and triangle; and prints a few letters, numbers, or words
    c. has a vocabulary of 2100 words; uses six- to eight-word sentences; names coins and names four or more colors; describes drawing; knows days of week and month; and can follow three commands in succession
 4. The functions served by these playmates are accomplished as the child gets older. Most children give up these friends when the group process becomes more important, usually when they enter school.
 5. a. jumping, running, climbing, swimming, skiing, skating, tricycles, scooter trucks, wagons, gym and sports equipment, sandboxes, wading pools, and winter sleds
    b. dress-up clothes, dolls, housekeeping toys, dollhouses, play-store toys, telephones, farm animals and equipment, trains, trucks, cars, planes, hand puppets, and doctor and nurse kits
 6. Because of improved gross motor skills and increasing independence, the preschooler is susceptible to injuries from such activities as playing in the street, riding a tricycle, chasing after balls, or forgetting safety regulations when crossing streets.
B.
 1. the social climate, type of guidance, and attitude toward the children that is fostered by the teacher or leader rather than whether or not structured learning is imposed
 2. a. Meet the director.
    b. Meet some of the caregivers or teachers.
    c. Systematically evaluate the facility in comparison with others.
    d. Observe the program in action.
 3. a. Present the idea of school as exciting and pleasurable.
    b. Talk to the child about the activities that he or she will participate in at school.
    c. Introduce the child to the teacher and familiarize him or her with the school.
    d. Provide the school with detailed information about the child's home environment, such as familiar routines, food preferences, etc.

C.
1. At about age 3 years, children are aware of anatomic differences between the sexes and are concerned with how the anatomy of the opposite sex works. They are really concerned about eliminative functions. This leads to physical exploration and questions to obtain more information.
2. a. This allows parents to identify the child's beliefs, and enables them not to give too much information.
   b. Although the child may forget information, information can be restated until the child absorbs and comprehends facts. This ensures no contradiction in information.
3. inability to fall asleep, bedtime fears, waking during the night, nightmares, prolonging bedtime through rituals
4. a. Accept the dream as real fear.
   b. Sit with the child; offer comfort, assurance, and a sense of protection.
   c. Avoid taking the child to the parents' own bed.
   d. Consider professional counseling for recurrent nightmares unresponsive to approaches above.
5. The American Academy of Pediatrics Committee on Nutrition recommends that by 5 years old, fatty acid consumption should be less than 10% of caloric intake. Parents should provide foods with less saturated fat (e.g., lowfat milk) and consider including soy-enriched foods.
6. the decreased quantity of food that the preschooler consumes
7. Advise parents to keep a weekly record of the child's diet in order to accurately estimate the intake of food at each meal. This should be evaluated at the end of a week's time. In most instances, the child has consumed more than the parent realizes.

Chapter 14

Review of Essential Concepts

1. a. recent exposure to a known case
   b. history of prodromal symptoms or evidence of constitutional symptoms
   c. history of previous immunizations
   d. previous history of having the disease
2. a. Child will not spread the infection to others.
   b. Child will not experience complications.
   c. Child will have minimal discomfort.
   d. Child and family will receive adequate emotional support.
3. a. prevention of disease through immunization
   b. control of the spread of disease
4. handwashing
5. a. those undergoing steroid or other immunosuppressive therapy
   b. those who have a generalized malignancy
   c. those who have an immunologic disorder
6. varicella (chicken pox), herpes zoster (shingles)
7. vitamin A supplements
8. a. cool baths
   b. use of lotions such as calamine
   c. avoiding overheating
   d. keeping nails short and smooth
   e. administering an antipruritic medication
9. a. 3
   b. 1
   c. 2
   d. 4
   e. 5
10. inflammation of the conjunctiva

11. a. obstruction of the nasolacrimal tear duct
    b. bacterial infection most frequent; also viral, allergic, and foreign body
12. b
13. a. keeping the eye clean
    b. properly administering ophthalmic medication
14. prevention of infection in other family members
15. a. aphthous stomatitis
    b. herpetic gingivostomatitis (HGS)
16. a. 1
    b. 2
    c. 1
    d. 2
17. giardiasis, pinworms
18. a. identification of the organism
    b. treatment of the infection
    c. prevention of initial infection or reinfection
19. preventive education of children and families regarding good hygiene and health habits
20. Giardia lamblia
21. Enterobiasis, pinworm
22. true
23. a. general irritability
    b. restlessness
    c. poor sleep
    d. bedwetting
    e. distractibility
    f. short attention span
24. tape test
25. It requires that certain potentially hazardous drugs and household products be sold in child-resistant containers.
26. a. Infants and toddlers explore their environment through oral experimentation.
    b. The sense of taste is less discriminating in small children, and many unpalatable substances are ingested.
    c. Toddlers and preschoolers are developing autonomy and initiative, which increases their curiosity.
    d. Imitation is a powerful motivator, especially when combined with a lack of awareness of danger.
27. a. assessment
    b. gastric decontamination
    c. prevention of recurrence
28. ipecac syrup
29. a. used in young infants in whom ipecac is contraindicated
    b. used if the patient is comatose or convulsing or requires a protected airway
    c. used if the ingested poison is rapidly absorbed
30. false
31. true
32. aspiration
33. Mucomyst
34. emesis; lavage; activated charcoal, or a cathartic
35. their level of hand to mouth activity is high
36. lead-based paint, soil
37. nervous
38. false
39. treatment actions
40. a. calcium disodium edetate (EDTA)
    b. succimer (chemet)
    c. British antilewisste (BAL)
41. prevention of initial or further exposure to lead

42. Child maltreatment
43. refers to a physical illness that one person fabricates or induces in another person; the perpetrator is seeking attention for themselves from medical staff.
44. a. parental characteristics
    b. characteristics of the child
    c. environmental characteristics
45. severely punished, more
46. a. incest
    b. molestation
    c. exhibitionism
    d. child pornography
    e. child prostitution
    f. pedophilia
47. a. Protect the child from further abuse.
    b. Support the child and family.
    c. The hospitalized child and family will be prepared for discharge.
    d. Prevent abuse.

Applying Critical Thinking to Nursing Practice

A.
 1. through a tape test or inspection of the anal area while the child sleeps
 2. a. Identify the parasite.
    b. Eradicate the organism.
    c. Prevent reinfection.
B.
 1. a. Obtain vital signs and initiate any needed respiratory and/or circulatory support; institute measures to reduce effects of shock; maintain respiratory function; anticipate and prepare for potential problems.
    b. Induce vomiting if indicated; administer antidotes; assist with gastric lavage; possible administration of activated charcoal; be aware of indications and contraindications for the various decontamination procedures.
    c. Discuss difficulties of constantly safeguarding young children; make a follow-up home visit for assessment of potential hazards; ask specific questions to isolate risk factors; emphasize proper storage of poisons.
 2. a. S
    b. S
    c. S
    d. A
C.
 1. decrease in intellectual functions, development of learning problems, and behavior problems
 2. to refer the child immediately for examination and lead screening
 3. a. 20-44
    b. 45-69
    c. 70
 4. a. Inject local anesthetic procaine with chelating drug.
    b. Rotate injection sites.
    c. Keep intake and output; monitor urinalysis and renal function. Implement seizure precautions.
 5. a. Wash child's hands and face before eating.
    b. Use cold water tap for drinking, cooking, and making formula.
    c. Do not store food in open cans, particularly if cans are imported.
    d. Do not use pottery or ceramic ware that was inadequately fired or is meant for decorative use.
    e. Make sure the child eats regular meals, since more lead is absorbed on an empty stomach.
    f. Make sure the child's diet contains plenty of iron and calcium and not too much fat.

D.

1. a. type of parenting received; negative relationship with own parents; social isolation; low self-esteem; no support system; with presence of concurrent stresses; inadequate knowledge of normal development; lack of knowledge of parenting skills
   b. temperament; position in the family; additional physical and/or emotional needs; activity level; illegitimacy; reminds parents of someone they dislike; prematurity; product of difficult delivery
   c. chronic stress from many sources
2. a. a thorough physical examination
   b. detailed history
3. Any five of the following are acceptable:
   Conflicting stories about the accident or injury
   Cause of injury blamed on sibling or other party
   An injury inconsistent with the history
   History inconsistent with the child's developmental level
   A complaint other than the obvious injury
   Inappropriate response of caregiver
   Inappropriate response of child
   Repeated visits to emergency facilities with injuries
4. a. risk for trauma related to characteristics of child, caregiver(s), environment
   b. fear/anxiety related to negative interpersonal interaction, repeated maltreatment, powerlessness, potential loss of parents
   c. altered parenting related to child, caregiver, or situational characteristics that precipitate abusive behavior
5. The record of the hospital admission or home visit may be important evidence of abuse in court proceedings.
6. a. Child experiences no further injury or neglect.
   b. Parents exhibit evidence of positive interaction with children.
   c. Parents demonstrate an understanding of normal expectations for their child.
7. The nurse must identify his or her own feelings in order to establish and maintain a therapeutic relationship with the child and the family—including the abusers.

Chapter 15

Review of Essential Concepts

1. beginning—shedding of deciduous teeth; ending—at puberty with the acquisition of permanent teeth
2. false
3. a. a decrease in head circumference in relation to standing height
   b. a decrease in waist circumference in relation to height
   c. an increase in leg length related to height
4. 12, 14
5. d
6. d
7. inferiority
8. true
9. c
10. true
11. conservation
12. the ability to group objects according to the attributes they share and place things in a sensible and logical order
13. true
14. d
15. b

16. family, peers
17. peer group
18. a. to appreciate the numerous and varied points of view that are represented in the peer group
    b. to become increasingly sensitive to the social norms and pressure of the peer group
    c. to form intimate friendships between same-sex peers
19. formalized groups, clubs
20. Bullying, peers
21. social, intellectual, and physical skill growth
22. a conscious awareness of a variety of self-perceptions, such as one's physical characteristics, abilities, values, self-ideals, and expectancies and one's idea of self in relation to others
23. family
24. teachers
25. latchkey children
26. lying, cheating, stealing
27. stomach pains or headaches, sleep problems, bedwetting, changes in eating habits, aggressive or stubborn behavior, reluctance to participate in activities, regression to earlier behaviors
28. a. 1
    b. 2
    c. 2
    d. 3
29. a. easy availability of high-calorie foods
    b. tendency toward more sedentary activities
30. true
31. a. physiologic aspects of human sexuality
    b. cultural and societal values
    c. his or her own attitudes, feelings, and biases about sexuality
32. true
33. true

Applying Critical Thinking to Nursing Practice

A.
1. a. falls at the 50th percentile
   b. falls at the 50th percentile
2. At Jimmy's stage of development, he needs and wants real achievement. When he has access to tasks that need to be done, and he is positively rewarded, he will be able to achieve a sense of industry and accomplishment.
3. Lying, cheating, and stealing are frequent occurrences in the young school-age child. Children of this age often have difficulty separating fact and fantasy. Parents need to teach them the difference. This will often disappear as they mature.

B.
1. The child needs to fit into a peer group and gain a sense of industry through individual and cooperative performance. It is necessary to move away from the familiar relationships of the family group to increase the scope of interpersonal interactions and explore the environment.
2. Identification with peers is a strong influence in the gaining of independence from parents. This is the first time that children are able to join in group activities with unrestrained enthusiasm and steady participation.
3. a. Educate the child regarding proper use of seat belts while a passenger in a vehicle.
   b. Maintain discipline while a passenger in a vehicle.
   c. Remind parents that the child should not ride in the bed of a pick-up truck.
   d. Teach the child how to be a safe pedestrian.
   e. Insist on wearing safety apparel (helmet when riding a bicycle, motorcycle, moped, or all-terrain vehicle).
4. a. Teach the child to swim.
   b. Teach basic rules of water safety.
   c. Teach children to select safe and supervised places to swim.

d. Teach the child to check sufficient water depth for diving.

e. Teach the child to swim with a companion.

f. Insist that the child use an approved flotation device in water or boats.

Chapter 16

Review of Essential Concepts

1. secondary sex characteristics, body growth
2. a. the maturational, hormonal, and growth processes that occur when the reproductive organs begin to function and secondary sex characteristics develop
   b. means "to grow into maturity" and is generally regarded as the psychologic, social, and maturational process initiated by the pubertal changes
3. hormonal activity
4. a. increased physical growth
   b. appearance and development of secondary sex characteristics
5. a. the external and internal organs that carry on the reproductive functions
   b. changes that occur throughout the body as a result of the hormonal changes
6. Estrogen, androgens
7. 10.5, 15; 12 years $9\frac{1}{2}$ months
8. testicular, pubic hair
9. growth spurt
10. a. 1
    b. 1
    c. 1
    d. 2
11. true
12. Sebaceous
13. true
14. b
15. group, personal or individual
16. when the individual is unable to formulate a satisfactory identity from the multiplicity of aspirations, roles, and identifications
17. peers, adults
18. mature, childlike
19. formal operations
20. a. can think beyond the present
    b. is capable of formal logic
    c. is capable of mentally manipulating more than two categories of variables at the same time
    d. is able to detect logical inconsistencies and can evaluate a system of values in a more analytic manner
    e. is able to differentiate the thoughts of others from his or her own
21. peer group
22. separate from their parents and become independent
23. 50%
24. same-sex
25. false
26. "Am I normal?"
27. health-damaging behaviors
28. true
29. a. poor dietary habits
    b. increased sedentary lifestyle
30. visual refractive difficulties

31. Any five of the following are acceptable:
    body image
    sexuality conflicts
    scholastic pressures
    competitive pressures
    relationship with parents
    relationship with siblings
    relationship with peers
    finances
    decisions about present and future roles
    career planning
    ideologic conflicts
32. true
33. physical injury
34. motor vehicle crashes
35. alcohol

Applying Critical Thinking to Nursing Practice

A.
1. a. between the 50th and 75th percentile
   b. at the 95th percentile
2. Nonlean body mass, primarily fat, increases in adolescence. Fatty tissue deposition is more pronounced in girls, particularly in the regions over the thighs, hips, buttocks, and breast tissue. While the 95th percentile is the top of the normal range, nutritional counseling to prevent additional weight gain and/or eating disorders should be instituted.

B.
1. A sense of group identity is essential to the later development of personal identity. Younger adolescents must resolve questions concerning relationships with a peer group before they are able to resolve questions about who they are in relation to the family and society.
2. a. wearing clothes, makeup, and hairstyles according to group criteria
   b. enjoying music and dancing that is exclusive to the age group
   c. using the same language
   d. conforming to the peer group rather than to the adult world
3. They serve as a strong support to the adolescent, individually and collectively, providing a sense of belonging and a feeling of strength and power. They form a transitional world between dependence and autonomy.

C.
1. Rapid physical growth, increased activity, and a propensity for staying up late tend to contribute to this.
2. a. exercise for growing muscles
   b. interactions with peers
   c. socially acceptable means to enjoy stimulation and conflict
3. This is a period when orthodontic appliances are usually worn, so it is important to provide instructions regarding use and care of the appliances and emphasize attention to toothbrushing.
4. The need for independence, coupled with the propensity for risk taking and feelings of indestructibility, makes the adolescent vulnerable. The need for peer approval often causes the adolescent to attempt hazardous feats.
5. a. motor vehicle accidents
   b. nonautomotive vehicle injuries
   c. firearms
   d. sports injuries
6. a. simple, correct explanations of body and sexual functions
   b. accurate information about menarche, pregnancy, contraception, masturbation
   c. the transmission, symptoms, and treatment of sexually transmitted diseases
   d. information about sexuality in the opposite sex and homosexuality

7. a. Begin with their present diet and actively involve them in the process.
   b. Respect their independence and give them opportunity to make their own selections and decisions.
   c. Adolescents will be more receptive to nutritional diet choices if linked to physical appearance.
   d. Provide straightforward information; talk with them, not at them; and listen carefully.

Chapter 17

Review of Essential Concepts

1. Epstein-Barr
2. a. headache
   b. malaise
   c. fatigue
   d. chilliness
   e. low-grade fever
   f. loss of appetite
   g. puffy eyes
3. Monospot
4. imitation of adult behavior, peer pressure, desire to imitate behaviors in movies, and a desire to control weight
5. false
6. personal and social
7. a. "Little League elbow"
   b. "tennis elbow"
   c. Osgood-Schlatter disease
8. repeated muscle contraction in repetitive weight-bearing sports
9. a. preparation and evaluation for activities
   b. prevention of injury
   c. treatment of injuries
   d. rehabilitation after injury
10. true
11. inadequate nutrition
12. a. short stature
    b. sexual infantilism
    c. amenorrhea
13. a. azoospermia
    b. defective development of secondary sex characteristics
14. false
15. prostaglandins
16. front, back
17. mass, testis
18. testicular self-examination
19. a. premature labor
    b. infants of low birth weight
    c. high neonatal mortality
    d. pregnancy-induced hypertension (PIH)
    e. iron deficiency anemia
    f. fetopelvic disproportion
    g. prolonged labor
20. suited to the individual
21. human papilloma virus (HPV), chlamydia
22. a. herpes progenitalis
    b. acquired immunodeficiency syndrome (HIV)

23. a. 4, 10
    b. 1, 7
    c. 2, 8
    d. 5, 9
    e. 3, 6
24. gonorrheal, chlamydial
25. effects on the reproductive system, such as acute abscess formation in the fallopian tubes, chronic pelvic pain, dyspareunia, formation of adhesions, and increased risk for ectopic pregnancy
26. a. all right
    b. not being blamed for the situation
27. a. the acute phase of disorganization of lifestyle
    b. the long-term reorganization process
28. avoid inflicting further stress on the victim
29. obese, 95th
30. a. hypothalamic
    b. hereditary
    c. metabolic
    d. social
    e. cultural
    f. psychologic
31. a. adipose cell theory
    b. set point theory
32. a. Modify the diet to provide loss of fat content without interfering with growth, normal activity, and psychologic well-being.
    b. Implement a regular exercise program.
    c. Modify eating behavior.
    d. Provide psychologic support.
33. motivation
34. a
35. false
36. Anorexia nervosa
37. 13
38. a. a relentless pursuit of thinness
    b. a fear of fatness
39. a. severe and profound weight loss
    b. secondary or primary amenorrhea
    c. bradycardia
    d. lowered body temperature
    e. decreased blood pressure
    f. cold intolerance
    g. dry skin and brittle nails
    h. appearance of lanugo hair
40. a. reinstitution of normal nutrition or reversal of malnutrition
    b. resolution of disturbed patterns of family interaction
    c. individual psychotherapy to correct deficits and distortions in psychological functioning
41. Bulimia
42. self-induced vomiting; diuretics and laxative abuse; enemas
43. a. those who purge
    b. those who don't purge
44. true
45. a. monitoring of fluid and electrolyte alterations
    b. observation for signs of cardiac complications
46. developmentally inappropriate degrees of inattention, impulsiveness, and hyperactivity

47. a. family education and counseling
    b. medication
    c. proper classroom placement
    d. environmental manipulation
    e. behavioral and/or psychotherapy for child
48. intentional or involuntary urination (usually nocturnal) in children beyond the age when voluntary bladder control should normally have been acquired
49. a. drugs
    b. bladder training
    c. restriction or elimination of fluids after evening meal
    d. interruption of sleep to void
    e. devices to establish a conditioned reflex response
50. repeated voluntary or involuntary passage of feces of normal or near-normal consistency into places not appropriate for that purpose according to the individual's own sociocultural setting
51. a. persistent reexperiencing of the traumatic event
    b. avoidance of stimuli associated with event or trauma
    c. numbing of general responsiveness and increased arousal
52. a. initial response
    b. mobilization of defense mechanisms
    c. coping
53. immediate return of the child to school
54. psychogenic
55. psychophysiologic disorder with a sudden onset that can usually be traced to a precipitating environmental event
56. false
57. a. predominantly sad facial expression with absence or diminished range of affective response
    b. solitary play, work, or tendency to be alone; disinterest in play
    c. withdrawal from previously enjoyed activities and relationships
    d. lowered grades in school; lack of interest in doing homework or achieving in school
    e. diminished motor activity; tiredness
    f. tearfulness or crying
    g. dependent and clinging or aggressive and disruptive
58. ego
59. true
60. a. Alcohol, central nervous
    b. Crack
    c. HIV, hepatitis B
    d. Methamphedamine
    e. Sniffing
61. function
62. true
63. a. preoccupation with thoughts about committing suicide and may be a precursor to suicide
    b. refers to all behaviors ranging from gestures to serious attempts to kill oneself
64. drug overdose
65. false
66. a. early recognition
    b. management
    c. prevention
67. recognition

Applying Critical Thinking to Nursing Practice

A.

1. on the basis of clinical manifestations, an absolute increase in atypical lymphocytes, a positive heterophil agglutination test, and a positive Monospot test
2. a. within 7 to 10 days
   b. within 2 to 4 weeks
   c. 2 to 3 months
3. a short course of oral penicillin, gargles, hot drinks, analgesic troches, analgesics including opioids
4. a. to relieve the symptoms
   b. to establish appropriate activities according to stage of disease and her interests

B.

1. rest or alteration of activities, physical therapy, and medication; alternative exercise should be used to help the athlete to maintain conditioning.
2. whether running provides both pleasure and physical benefits for him at the present time and perhaps into adulthood
3. a. Ensure that safety measures are utilized.
   b. Require proper warmup and cool-down activities.
   c. Establish appropriate training requirements for safe participation.
   d. Ensure that protective equipment is utilized.

C.

1. stress, changes in environment, weight changes, hyperandrogenism, eating disorders, and exercise-induced amenorrhea
2. nonsteroidal antiinflammatory drugs
3. a. Teach information about these diseases in sex education classes.
   b. Encourage abstinence or postponement of sexual intercourse; encourage condom use; advise to take hepatitis B vaccination.
   c. Decrease the medical and psychologic effects through support groups.

D.

1. because it is obvious to others, is difficult to treat, and has long-term effects on psychologic and physical health status
2. a. altered nutrition, more than body requirements, related to dysfunctional eating patterns, hereditary factors
   b. activity intolerance related to sedentary lifestyle, physical bulk
   c. ineffective individual coping related to little or no exercise, poor nutrition, personal vulnerability
   d. self-esteem disturbance related to perception of physical appearance, internalization, or negative feedback
   e. altered family processes related to management of child who is obese
3. a. The child will follow a diet that provides loss of fat content without interfering with growth, normal activity, and psychologic well-being.
   b. The child will engage in a regular exercise program.
   c. The child will modify his or her eating behavior.
   d. The child and family will receive psychologic support.

E.

1. The weight loss may be triggered by an adolescent crisis such as the onset of menstruation or a traumatic interpersonal incident that precipitates dieting that continues out of control.
2. a. the current emphasis on slimness
   b. increased family stress, adolescent feels lack of personal control
3. a. B
   b. A, B
   c. A
   d. A
   e. B
   f. A
   g. B

F.

1. Ingestion of drugs prescribed for parents is a common method of a suicide attempt.
2. a disturbed family situation; parental loss; family history of suicide, depression, substance abuse, or emotional disturbance; child abuse or neglect; unavailable parents; poor communication and isolation within the family; family conflict; unrealistically high parental expectations or parental indifference with low expectations
3. family support and counseling, have Michelle sign a contract that she will not attempt another suicide, and individual counseling

Chapter 18

Review of Essential Concepts

1. children who have or are at increased risk for a chronic physical, developmental, behavioral, or emotional condition and who also require health and related services of a type or amount beyond that generally required by children
2. a. 3
   b. 1
   c. 4
   d. 2
3. a. focus on the child's developmental age rather than chronologic age or diagnosis; emphasizes child's abilities and strengths
   b. a philosophy of care that recognizes the family as the constant in a child's life
4. a. Normalize the life of a child with special needs in a family and community setting.
   b. Minimize the disruptive impact of the child's condition on the family.
   c. Foster the child's maximum growth and development.
5. Mainstreaming
6. a. Accept the child's condition.
   b. Manage the child's condition on a day-to-day basis.
   c. Meet the child's normal developmental needs.
   d. Meet the developmental needs of other family members.
   e. Cope with ongoing stress and periodic crises.
   f. Assist family members to manage their feelings.
   g. Educate others about the child's condition.
   h. Establish a support system.
7. true
8. Any three of the following are acceptable:
   Value each child individually and avoid comparisons.
   Help siblings see differences and similarities between themselves and the child with special needs.
   Teach siblings ways to interact with the child.
   Seek to be fair in terms of discipline, attention, and resources.
   Let siblings settle their own differences.
   Legitimize reasonable anger.
   Respect a sibling's reluctance to be with or to include the child with special needs in activities.
9. Empowerment
10. a. shock and denial
    b. adjustment
    c. reintegration and acknowledgment
11. a. guilt
    b. self-accusation
    c. bitterness
    d. anger

12. a. The parents fear letting the child achieve any new skill, they avoid all discipline, and they cater to every desire to prevent frustration.
    b. The parents detach themselves emotionally from the child but usually provide adequate physical care or constantly nag and scold the child.
    c. The parents act as if the disorder does not exist or attempt to have the child overcompensate for it.
    d. The parents place necessary and realistic restrictions on the child, encourage self-care activities, and promote reasonable physical and social abilities.
13. feeling of sorrow and loss that recurs in waves over time
14. This concept considers the issues related to caring for and living with the child in relation to the family's resources and ability to cope.
15. a. the child's developmental level
    b. temperament
    c. available coping mechanisms
    d. the reactions of family members or significant others
    e. the condition itself
16. true
17. a. develops competence and optimism
    b. feels different and withdraws
    c. is irritable, moody, and acts out
    d. complies with treatment
    e. seeks support
18. a. available support system
    b. perception of the illness/disability
    c. coping mechanisms
    d. available resources
    e. concurrent stresses
19. a. denial
    b. guilt
    c. anger
20. a. Observe the child's responses to the disorder, ability to function, and adaptive behaviors within the environment.
    b. Explore the child's own understanding of the nature of this illness or condition.
    c. Provide support while the child learns to cope with his or her feelings.
21. a. preparation
    b. participation
    c. sharing
    d. control
    e. expectation
22. self-care abilities in both activities of daily living and the medical regimen
23. provides a child with boundaries on which to test out his or her behavior; teaches socially acceptable behavior
24. realistic future goals
25. the achievement of the best possible quality of life for patients and their families
26. false
27. separation from parents
28. The goal is for children to live life to the fullest without pain, with choices and dignity, in the familiar environment of their home and with the support of their family.
29. a. fear of pain and suffering
    b. fear of dying alone (child) or of not being present when the child dies (parent)
    c. fear of actual death
30. guilty, shameful
31. a. sensations of somatic distress
    b. preoccupation with image of the deceased
    c. feelings of guilt
    d. feelings of hostility
    e. loss of usual patterns of conduct

32. take years
33. a. Maintain good general health.
    b. Develop well-rounded interests.
    c. Use distance techniques.
    d. Develop and utilize professional and personal support systems.
    e. Cultivate the capacity for empathy.
    f. Focus on positive aspects of the caregiver role.
    g. Base nursing interventions on sound theory and empirical observations.

Applying Critical Thinking to Nursing Practice

A.
1. a. care now focused on the child's developmental age rather than chronologic age
    b. care now focused on family-centered care
    c. increased use of the principle of normalization
    d. tend toward mainstreaming, or integrating children with special needs into a regular classroom
2. a. Using the developmental approach emphasizes the child's abilities and strengths rather than his or her disability. Under the developmental model, attention is directed to the child's functional development, changes, and adaptation to the environment.
    b. Families are supported in their natural caregiving and decision-making roles by building on their unique strengths as individuals and families.
    c. By applying the principles of normalization, the environment for the child is "normalized" and "humanized."
    d. The school has now become an essential component of the child's overall physical, intellectual, and social development.

B.
1. a. This is a period of intense emotion and is characterized by shock, disbelief, and sometimes denial, especially if the disorder is not obvious.
    b. This follows shock and is usually characterized by an open admission that the condition exists. This stage is manifested by several responses such as guilt and anger.
    c. This stage is characterized by realistic expectations for the child and reintegration of family life, with the child's condition in proper perspective. The family also broadens its activities to include relationships outside the home, with the child being an acceptable and participating member of the group.
2. a. shopping for physicians
    b. attributing the symptoms of the actual illness to a minor condition
    c. refusal to believe the diagnostic tests
    d. delay in agreeing to treatment
    e. acting very happy and optimistic despite the revealed diagnosis
    f. refusing to tell or talk to anyone about the condition
    g. insisting that no one is telling the truth regardless of others' attempts to do so
    h. denying the reason for admission
    i. asking no questions about the diagnosis, treatment, or prognosis
3. a. It allows parents to distance themselves from the onslaught of a tremendous emotional impact and to collect and mobilize their energies toward goal-directed problem-solving behaviors.
    b. It allows the child to maintain hope in the face of overwhelming odds.
4. Assure her that the sister's behavior is understandable in light of her sibling's illness. She is experiencing many conflicting feelings because of the focus of attention on the ill child and the loss of the sibling interaction with the ill child. Try to reserve a few minutes each day to spend focused time with the healthy child. Include the healthy child in activities involving care of the ill child when possible.

C.
1. a. status of the marital relationship
    b. alternate support systems
    c. ability to communicate
2. This aids in evaluating the individual's ability to cope with various aspects of the crisis and identifies possible areas for intervention.

3. a. develops competence and optimism
   b. complies with treatment
   c. seeks support
4. a. Receive support at the time of diagnosis.
   b. Accept the family's emotional reactions.
   c. Support the family's coping methods.
   d. Educate about the disorder and general health care.
   e. Establish an environment of normalization for the child.
   f. Establish realistic future goals.
5. Parents verbalize feelings and concerns regarding implications of the disease. Family demonstrates an attitude of acceptance and adjustment.

D.
1. a. They see death as a departure, a kind of sleep.
   b. They may recognize the fact of physical death but do not separate it from living abilities.
   c. They view death as temporary and gradual; life and death can change places with each other.
   d. They have no understanding of the universality and inevitability of death.
2. as punishment for his or her thoughts or actions
3. 9, 10
4. a. Help parents deal with their feelings, allowing them more emotional reserve to meet the needs of their children.
   b. Avoid alliances with either the parent or the child.
   c. Structure the hospital admission to allow for maximum self-control and independence.
   d. Answer the adolescent's questions honestly, treating him or her as a mature individual and respecting his or her need for privacy, solitude, and personal expression of emotions.
   e. Help parents understand their child's reactions to death/dying.

E.
1. a. Support the child during the terminal phase.
   b. Provide physical comfort at time of dying.
   c. Provide emotional support at time of dying.
2. a. Child expresses feelings freely.
   b. Child demonstrates an understanding of symptoms.
3. d

Chapter 19

Review of Essential Concepts

1. The definition of mental retardation in children is comprised of three components that assess intellectual functioning, functional strengths and weaknesses, and age at time of diagnosis (less than 18 years of age). Intellectual functioning is measured by intellectual quotient (IQ) and is 70-75 or below. In addition, the child must demonstrate functional impairment in at least 2 of 10 different adaptive skill areas.
2. after a period of suspicion by professionals and/or the family that the child's developmental progress is delayed
3. a. intellectual functioning and adaptive skills
   b. psychologic/emotional considerations
   c. physical health/etiology considerations
   d. environmental considerations
4. educable mentally retarded
5. a. mild
   b. moderate
   c. severe
   d. profound

6. a. genetic
   b. biochemical
   c. infectious
7. Early intervention programs
8. This act encourages local departments of education to provide early intervention services and requires them to provide educational opportunities for all children with disabilities from 0 to 21 years of age.
9. a. A task analysis of the individual steps needed to master a skill must be done before teaching.
   b. Observe the child to determine what skills are possessed and the child's developmental readiness to learn the task.
10. recreational, educational
11. Safety
12. simple, consistently, appropriate
13. Provide practical sexual information and a well-defined, concrete code of conduct regarding sexuality.
14. 21
15. through presence of clinical manifestations and a chromosomal analysis
16. hypotonicity of chest and abdominal muscles and dysfunction of immune system
17. cardiac
18. fragile X
19. a. indicates disability that may range in severity from mild to profound and includes the subsets of deaf and hard-of-hearing
   b. refers to a person whose hearing disability precludes successful processing of linguistic information through audition, with or without a hearing aid
   c. a person who, generally with the use of a hearing aid, has residual hearing sufficient to enable successful processing of linguistic information through audition
20. a. family history
   b. anatomic malformation of head or neck
   c. low birth weight
   d. severe perinatal asphyxia
   e. perinatal infection (cytomegalovirus, rubella, herpes, syphilis, toxoplasmosis, bacterial meningitis)
   f. chronic ear infection
   g. cerebral palsy
   h. Down syndrome
   i. ototoxic drugs
21. a. an inability to express ideas in any form, either written or verbal
   b. the inability to interpret sound correctly
   c. difficulty in processing details or discriminating among sounds
22. decibels
23. acoustic feedback
24. hearing aid
25. Cochlear implants; earliest, 18
26. when there is visual acuity of 20/200 or less and/or a visual field of 20 degrees or less in the better eye
27. Refractive errors
28. true
29. a. 2, 4, 8
   b. 1, 7, 10
   c. 5, 9
   d. 3, 6
30. This is a reduced visual acuity in one eye. This results when one eye does not receive sufficient stimulation, and the brain suppresses the less intense image. It is also referred to as "lazy eye."
31. Strabismus
32. When there is malalignment, the eyes see two separate images (diplopia). Because the brain suppresses the images from the weaker or deviating eye, amblyopia can result.
33. esotropia

34. a. an opacity of the crystalline lens
    b. a condition in which intraocular pressure is increased, causing pressure on the optic nerve and eventually atrophy and blindness
35. because motor development is very dependent on sight
36. loss of sight and hearing
37. They interfere with the normal sequence of physical, intellectual, and psychosocial growth.
38. Retinoblastoma
39. cat's eye reflex
40. 90%
41. b

Applying Critical Thinking to Nursing Practice

A.
1. optimum medical care
2. a. promoting the child's optimum growth and development potential
   b. promoting the child's optimum socialization
3. a. developmental age of child
   b. special devices used by child
   c. effective measures of limit setting
   d. unusual or favorite routines
   e. any behaviors that might require intervention
   f. functional level of eating and playing
4. a. altered growth and development related to impaired cognitive functioning
   b. altered family processes related to having a child with mental retardation
5. to encourage successful attainment of goals and self-esteem
6. a. Family identifies realistic goals for future care of the child.
   b. Family avails themselves of supportive services.

B.
1. a. ensuring that the parents are informed as soon as possible following the birth of the child
   b. encouraging parents to be together at this time to emotionally support each other
   c. providing parents with written material concerning the syndrome
   d. discussing with parents the benefits of home care versus residential placement
2. a. hypertonicity of muscles
   b. hyperextensibility of joints
   c. decreased muscle tone causing respiratory dysfunction
   d. protruding tongue
   e. decreased muscle tone, causing decreased gastric motility, predisposing child to constipation
   f. rough and dry skin, and prone to cracking and infection

C.
1. a. Treat existing ear infections and prevent recurrences; encourage periodic auditory testing for children at risk; stress the need for routine immunizations; administer ototoxic agents cautiously; counsel pregnant women regarding the necessity of early prenatal care; prevent exposure to excessive noise.
   b. Screen all children for auditory function; observe for behaviors that indicate a hearing loss.
2. a. lack of startle reflex to a loud sound; failure to be awakened by loud environmental noises; failure to localize a source of sound by 6 months of age; absence of babble or inflections in voice by age 7 months; general indifference to sound; lack of response to the spoken word; response to loud noises as opposed to the voice
   b. use of gestures rather than verbalization; failure to develop intelligible speech by age 24 months; monotone and unintelligible speech; head banging, foot stamping; yelling or screeching to express pleasure; asking to have statements repeated; responding more to facial expression; avoidance of social interaction; suspicious alertness; irritable at not making himself or herself understood; shyness, timidity, withdrawal; appears dreamy and in world of his or her own

3. a. Enhance achievement of optimum independence level for age.
    b. Provide opportunity to participate in activities for play and socialization.
    c. Coordinate the opportunity to provide educational opportunities within a regular classroom.
D.
  1. a. identifying children who by virtue of their history are at risk
      b. observing for behaviors that indicate a vision loss
      c. screening all children for visual acuity and signs of other ocular disorders such as strabismus
  2. a. Support and educate the child and family.
      b. Parent-child attachment will develop.
      c. Promote the child's optimum development.
      d. Child will receive appropriate care during hospitalization.
  3. a. Help parents identify clues other than eye contact from the infant that signify communication.
      b. Encourage parents to show affection using nonvisual methods, such as talking, reading, cuddling, or walking the child.
E.
  1. Show them a picture of a child with an eye prosthesis. Prepare them for the appearance of the wound. Within 3 weeks the child will be fitted for a prosthesis, and the facial appearance will return to normal. Care of the socket is minimal and easily accomplished.
  2. Seek genetic counseling for themselves and for the child after he or she reaches puberty.
F.
  1. mentally retarded
  2. a. promote positive reinforcement
      b. increase social awareness of others
      c. teach verbal communication skills
      d. decrease unacceptable behavior

Chapter 20

Review of Essential Concepts

1. life, family
2. cost
3. family caregiver
4. a. lack of pediatric training in some nursing programs
    b. increased acuity of home care patients
    c. increased pay for nurses working in acute care settings
5. multidisciplinary, family
6. false
7. trial; pass
8. a. meeting the family
    b. helping the family assess their preparedness and the preparedness of the home environment
    c. discussing the arrangement of the child's equipment at home
    d. reinforcing prior discharge teaching
    e. implementing additional teaching that is necessary
9. care coordination
10. ensuring continuity for the child and family across hospital, home, educational, therapeutic, and other settings
11. a. Reduce the complexity of care for the child.
    b. Reduce fragmentation of care.
    c. Decrease the burden of care for the family.
12. family's, family's
13. technical, adapt

14. a. demonstrates flexibility in skills and case management
    b. recognizes that the nurse is a guest in the home
    c. respects family culture and adapts appropriately
    d. works as an interdisciplinary team member
    e. demonstrates expertise in pediatric care
15. increasing, fewer
16. values
17. recognition that the family is the constant in the child's life, while the service systems and personnel within those systems fluctuate
18. true
19. a. racial
    b. ethnic
    c. cultural
    d. spiritual
    e. socioeconomic
20. family empowerment
21. collaboration
22. invasive, confidentiality
23. parental
24. family, family
25. priorities
26. child, family, professionals
27. development
28. a. initial and periodic assessment
    b. planning
    c. referrals for further assessment or therapeutic services
    d. interventions that address normalization issues and self-care
29. a. child's developmental age
    b. level of interest
    c. physical ability
    d. parental comfort and support
30. age-appropriate
31. individual family service plan
32. telephone, electric
33. emergency, parents
34. false
35. night
36. strengths, experience
37. accepted

Applying Critical Thinking to Nursing Practice

A.
  1. a. Include the family in the discharge planning process.
     b. Negotiate with the insurance company for more extensive home care hours.
     c. Involve the home care agency early to promote continuity and a smooth transition.
     d. Address health and community services that may need to be mobilized.
     e. Develop comprehensive written home care instructions.
     f. Have both parents learn and demonstrate all aspects of the child's care in the hospital.
  2. a. providing an in-hospital trial period during which the parents provide total care for Jonathan
     b. arranging for the parents to take him home on a day pass with the home care nurse present prior to making final discharge plans
  3. a. reinforcing the discharge teaching
     b. implementing any other teaching that is necessary

4. a. medical, nursing, and health maintenance needs of the child
   b. financial, psychosocial, and educational issues of the child and family

B.
 1. from the child's record
 2. to respect their privacy
 3. a. The nurse should respect parental preferences.
    b. A home care supervisor or case manager should be contacted for help with problem solving.
    c. The nurse should ask the parents to negotiate the change with the physician, since the nurse must follow the written medical orders.
 4. a. home as familiar
    b. home as protector, the location of everyday experiences related to time, space, and one's social life
    c. home as protector—privacy, safety, and identity may be preserved in the environment of the home

C.
 1. a. the extent to which the child is involved in his care
    b. modification in equipment and/or techniques for daily activities that promote self-care
    c. use of toys or other means to teach child self-care
 2. a. all medications, needles, syringes, and contaminated materials securely stored well out of reach of curious hands
    b. childproofing control panels for ventilators, pumps, monitors, and other equipment by use of clear plastic tape
    c. special lockout switches on medical equipment
    d. electrical cords short and out of reach; safety covers on any open outlets
    e. when not in use, equipment should be unplugged, and any wires should be stored out of reach

Chapter 21

Review of Essential Concepts

1. a. stress represents a change from usual state of health and environmental routine
   b. children have a limited number of coping mechanisms to deal with the stressors of these experiences
2. a. developmental age
   b. previous experience with illness, separation, or hospitalization
   c. innate and acquired coping skills
   d. seriousness of diagnosis
   e. available support system
3. separation
4. protest, despair, detachment (or denial)
5. peers
6. a. physical restriction
   b. altered routine or rituals
   c. dependency
7. a. 1
   b. 2
   c. 2
   d. 1
   e. 3
   f. 4
   g. 1
   h. 4
   i. 3
   j. 2

8. a. true
   b. false
   c. true
   d. false
   e. true
   f. true
   g. false
9. a. "difficult" temperament
   b. poor child-parent relationship
   c. age (especially between 6 months and 5 years)
   d. male gender
   e. below-average intelligence
   f. multiple and continuing stresses
10. a. disbelief
    b. anger, guilt
    c. fear, anxiety, frustration
    d. depression
11. loneliness, fear, worry, anger, resentment, jealousy, and guilt
12. Fear of the unknown (fantasy) exceeds fear of the known.
13. a. child's growth and development
    b. psychosocial needs
    c. educational needs
    d. cultural background
    e. effects of illness on the child's family or guardian
14. nursing process
15. separation
16. family-centered
17. a. separation
    b. physical restriction
    c. changed routines
    d. enforced dependency
    e. magical thinking
18. a. Promote freedom of movement.
    b. Maintain the child's routine.
    c. Encourage independence.
    d. Promote understanding.
19. false
20. Agency for Health Care Policy and Research
21. pain is whatever the experiencing person says it is, existing whenever the person says it does
22. a. Infants do not feel pain.
    b. Children tolerate pain better than adults do.
    c. Children cannot tell where they hurt.
    d. Children always tell the truth about their pain.
    e. Children become accustomed to pain or painful procedures.
    f. Behavioral manifestations of pain reflect pain intensity.
    g. Narcotics are more dangerous drugs for children than they are for adults.
23. a. a physiologic state in which abrupt cessation of the opioid, or administration of an opioid antagonist, results in a withdrawal syndrome
    b. a form of neuroadaptation to the effects of chronically administered opioids
    c. characterized by a persistent pattern of dysfunctional opioid use
24. a. Question the child.
    b. Use pain rating scales.
    c. Evaluate behavior and physiologic changes.
    d. Secure parents' involvement.
    e. Take cause of pain into account.
    f. Take action and evaluate results.

25. a. FACES scale
    b. Oucher
    c. poker chip tool
    d. word graphic rating scale
    e. numeric scale
    f. visual analogue scale
    g. color tool
26. a. Objective Pain Score (OPS)
    b. Children's Hospital of Eastern Ontario Pain Scale (CHEOPS)
    c. Nurses Assessment of Pain Inventory (NAPI)
    d. Behavioral Pain Score (BPS)
    e. Modified Behavioral Pain Scale (MBPS)
    f. Riley Infant Pain Scale (RIPS)
    g. FLACC Postoperative Pain Tool
27. distraction, relaxation, guided imagery, positive self-talk, thought stopping, cutaneous stimulation, and behavioral contracting
28. a. right drug
    b. right dose
    c. right route
    d. right time
29. Meperidine (Demerol)
30. potentiators
31. Demerol, Phenergan, and Thorazine
32. adjuvant analgesics, coanalgesics
33. equal analgesic effect between various routes of administration
34. patient-controlled analgesia (PCA)
35. epidural
36. eutectic mixture of local anesthetics
37. around-the-clock (ATC)
38. respiratory depression
39. constipation
40. work
41. a. 4
    b. 1
    c. 2
    d. 3
42. a. Family will participate in the child's care to the extent they desire.
    b. Family will receive support.
    c. Family will be informed of the child's care.
    d. Family will be prepared for discharge and home care.
43. a. minimization of the stressors of hospitalization
    b. reduced chance of infection
    c. cost savings
44. a. physical stressors
    b. environmental stressors
    c. psychologic stressors
    d. social stressors

Applying Critical Thinking to Nursing Practice

A.
 1. protest
 2. Any one of the following interventions is acceptable:
    Allow the child to cry.
    Provide support through physical presence in the room even when the child rejects strangers.

Acknowledge to the child that it is all right to miss his parents and it is all right to cry.

Encourage the parents to stay with the child as much as possible.

Parents should let the child know when they are leaving.

Parents should bring favorite articles from home to comfort the child.

B.

1. Any one of the following interventions is acceptable:

   Talk about the child's parents frequently.

   Encourage the child to talk about and remember family members or pets.

   Stress significance of parents and siblings' visits, telephone calls, or letters.

2. Any of the following interventions are acceptable:

   Use the minimum amount of restraint of physical activity.

   Set schedules and routines as close to that of the child as possible.

   Decrease dependency of the child by allowing her to do things for herself and allowing her to make decisions.

C.

1. a. encouraging parents to participate
   b. providing support to family members
   c. supplying information
   d. preparing for discharge and home care

2. Select three of the following:

   Respect parental rights.

   Convey an attitude of respectful caring for both child and family.

   Support and emphasize the family's strengths and abilities.

   Provide feedback and praise.

   Refer to other professionals for additional support.

3. Select three of the following:

   Recognize that family members know the child best and are "cued in" to the child's needs.

   Welcome unlimited family presence.

   Encourage family to bring other significant family members to visit.

   Encourage family to provide the child with significant but manageable items from home.

   Arrange for family members to have a meal together.

4. large puzzles, blocks, dress-up materials, puppets, scissors and paper, and crayons

5. a. Family demonstrates procedures needed to care for child in the home.
   b. Family is aware of how to seek help.

D.

1. a. Take a nursing admission history.
   b. Perform a physical assessment.
   c. Assess variables influencing placement of the child on the unit.

2. a. FACES
   b. Oucher
   c. Poker chip tool
   d. numeric scale
   e. visual analogue scale
   f. color tool

3. "around the clock" to avoid low plasma levels

4. a. respiratory depression
   b. constipation

Chapter 22

Review of Essential Concepts

1. the legal and ethical requirement that the patient clearly, fully, and completely understand the medical treatment to be performed and all risks of treatment and nontreatment before giving informed consent
2. a. The person must be capable of giving consent, must be over the age of majority, and must be considered competent.
   b. The person must receive the information needed to make an intelligent decision.
   c. The person must act voluntarily when exercising freedom of choice without force, fraud, deceit, duress, or other forms of constraint or coercion.
3. a. one who has attained the specific age at which a minor is permitted to give consent even though he or she is not technically an adult
   b. one who is legally under the age of majority but is recognized as having the legal capacity of an adult under circumstances prescribed by law (for example, marriage, pregnancy, etc.)
4. preparation
5. a. child's developmental level
   b. child's cognitive ability
   c. child's temperament
   d. child's existing coping strategies
   e. child's previous experiences
6. false
7. a. expect success
   b. involve the child
   c. provide distraction
   d. allow expression of feelings
8. a. teach
   b. express feelings
   c. achieve a therapeutic goal
9. a. 3
   b. 2
   c. 1
   d. 4
10. true
11. 2
12. a. Guard the patient's safety and welfare.
    b. Minimize physical discomfort or pain.
    c. Minimize negative psychologic responses to treatment by providing analgesia and maximize the potential for amnesia.
    d. Control behavior.
    e. Return the patient to a state in which safe discharge, as determined by recognized criteria, is possible.
13. the extent to which the patient's behavior coincides with the prescribed regimen
14. a. clinical judgment
    b. self-reporting
    c. direct observation
    d. monitoring appointments
    e. monitoring therapeutic response
    f. pill counts
    g. chemical assay
15. a. organizational strategies
    b. educational strategies
    c. treatment strategies
    d. behavioral strategies

16. amount, tissue damage
17. widely spaced teeth, pomade
18. avoided, osmotic
19. a. vomiting or diarrhea
    b. decrease in appetite
    c. abdominal cramping or distention
    d. absence of bowel sounds
    e. dehydration or weight loss
20. elevated temperature
21. a. 3
    b. 1
    c. 2
22. antipyretics
23. Acetaminophen
24. a. C
    b. I
    c. C
    d. C
    e. I
25. a. synthesize the major features of universal precautions and body substance isolation; designed for use with all patients, especially those who are undiagnosed
    b. used for patients known or suspected to be infected with epidemiologically important pathogens for which additional precautions beyond standard precautions are needed to interrupt transmission in hospitals
26. airborne, droplet, contact
27. Handwashing
28. time-out
29. age, condition, destination
30. Restraints, physician's
31. glucose, ketones, protein, blood, bilirubin, urobilinogen, nitrates, potassium, creatinine, and urea
32. Catheterization, sterile
33. necrotizing osteochondritis
34. body weight
35. a. vastus lateralis muscle
    b. ventrogluteal muscle
36. walking, 1
37. a. amount of drug to be administered
    b. minimum dilution of drug
    c. type of solution in which drug can be diluted
    d. length of time over which drug can be safely administered
    e. rate of infusion that child and vessels can tolerate safely
    f. IV tubing volume capacity
    g. time that this or another drug is to be administered
    h. compatibility of all drugs that child is receiving intravenously
38. Peripheral venous access devices
39. a. short-term or nontunneled catheters
    b. peripherally inserted central catheter (PICC)
    c. long-term central VADs (ports)
40. weighed; One, one
41. fluids, complications
42. they can accurately infuse fluids
43. retina, lungs
44. a. pulse oximetry
    b. transcutaneous monitoring (TCM)

45. a. effective in depositing medication directly into the airway
    b. avoids the systemic side effects of certain drugs
    c. reduces the amount of drug necessary to achieve the desired effect
46. true
47. chest physiotherapy
48. humidified
49. increased heart rate; a rise in respiratory effort; a drop in O_2 saturation; cyanosis; or an increase in the positive inspiratory pressure (PIP) on the ventilator
50. only as often as necessary to keep the tube patent
51. pH
52. MIC-KEY, Bard Button, Gastroport
53. protein, glucose
54. superior vena cava, innominate, intrathoracic subclavian veins
55. rapid fluid shift and fluid overload
56. a. Osmotic effect of the enema may produce diarrhea, which can lead to metabolic acidosis.
    b. Extreme hyperphosphatemia, hypernatremia, hypocalcemia can occur, which may lead to neuromuscular irritability and coma.
57. peristomal skin

Applying Critical Thinking to Nursing Practice

A.
  1. a. Patient will give fully informed consent and sign appropriate documents.
     b. Patient will receive proper hygiene measures.
     c. Patient will receive proper preparation.
     d. Patient will experience no complications.
     e. Patient will experience no injury.
  2. a. instituting preoperative teaching
     b. orienting child to strange surroundings
     c. explaining where parents will be while child is in operating room
     d. having someone stay with child
  3. Child exhibits no evidence of complications.
B.
  1. Measure the rectal temperature 30 minutes after the antipyretic is given to assess whether the temperature is lowered.
  2. Use minimal clothing, expose skin to air, reduce room temperature, increase air circulation, and administer cool applications to the skin.
  3. crib sides
C.
  1. a. increasing nutritional and fluid intake
     b. how to decrease elevated temperature
     c. safety concerns
     d. infection control
     e. play
  2. Toys must be safe and appropriate to child's developmental level and condition.
D.
  1. a. Allow Daniel to see that there is always someone nearby.
     b. Allow him to have a favorite toy inside the tent.
     c. If he is well enough, remove Daniel from the tent for feeding and bathing.
  2. This minimizes the chance of vomiting and aspiration.
  3. You would auscultate the chest before treatment and then after treatment to hear whether the chest sounds clearer.

E.
1. a. keeping skin around stoma clean and dry
   b. maintaining aseptic technique
   c. suctioning as needed
   d. keeping an extra tracheostomy set at the bedside
   e. checking patency of tube frequently by auscultation of the chest
   f. monitoring the child for problems such as pallor, cyanosis, changes in pulse and/or blood pressure, and bleeding around the site
2. noisy breathing, bubbling, or coughing
3. to prevent hypoxia

F.
1. a. because this entry causes less distress (since infants are obligatory nose breathers) and helps stimulate sucking
   b. so that the fluid and electrolyte balance won't be upset by removing fluids and electrolytes
   c. because of possible damage to the nostril
   d. to clear formula from the tube and prevent souring
   e. to minimize the possibility of regurgitation and aspiration
2. a. attaching a syringe to the feeding tube and attempting to aspirate stomach contents; checking pH; returning contents to stomach
   b. injecting 0.5 ml of air into the tube with the syringe, while listening with a stethoscope to the stomach area for sounds of gurgling or growling; withdrawing air
3. a. Return residual aspirated fluid to the stomach.
   b. Provide a pacifier during feeding.

Chapter 23

Review of Essential Concepts

1. a. age of the child
   b. the season
   c. living conditions
   d. preexisting medical problems
2. The diameter of the respiratory tract is smaller and therefore subject to narrowing from edematous mucous membranes and increased production of secretions.
3. a. true
   b. true
   c. true
   d. false
   e. true
   f. false
   g. true
4. a. Child will exhibit normal respiratory effort.
   b. Child will receive adequate rest.
   c. Child will remain comfortable.
   d. Child will not spread primary infection to others.
   e. Child's temperature will remain within normal limits.
   f. Child will maintain normal hydration and adequate nutrition.
   g. Child will experience no complications.
   h. Child and family will receive information, especially concerning home care, and support.
5. Saline nose drops
6. symptomatic
7. ineffective
8. group A β-hemolytic streptococci (GABHS)

9. throat culture
10. penicillin or other antibiotic for at least 10 days
11. to filter and protect the respiratory and the alimentary tracts from invasion by pathogenic organisms and play a role in antibody formation
12. palatine tonsils
13. adenoids
14. inflammation; swallowing, breathing
15. blockage of the nares, which interferes with air passage from nose to throat; as a result, child breathes through the mouth
16. a. there is malignancy and obstruction of the airway
    b. the child has hypertrophied adenoids that obstruct nasal breathing
    c. there are three or more infections of tonsils and/or adenoids per year despite adequate medical therapy
17. 24 hours
18. hemorrhage
19. frequent swallowing
20. aspirin
21. a. an inflammation of the middle ear without reference to etiology or pathogenesis
    b. a rapid and short onset of signs and symptoms lasting approximately 3 weeks
    c. an inflammation of the middle ear in which a collection of fluid is present in the middle ear space
    d. middle ear effusion that persists beyond 3 months
22. *Streptococcus pneumoniae, Hemophilus influenzae, Moraxella catarrhalis*
23. bulging or full, opacified, or very reddened immobile membrane
24. oral amoxicillin
25. hearing loss
26. tympanostomy tubes
27. the primary anatomic area affected
28. a. maintaining an airway
    b. providing for adequate respiratory exchange
29. to decrease edema of the respiratory tract
30. an obstructive inflammatory process of the epiglottis
31. edematous
32. it could precipitate a spasm of the epiglottis and complete obstruction of the airway
33. respiratory syncytial virus (RSV)
34. Bronchiole mucosa swells and lumina are filled with mucus and exudate.
    The walls of bronchi and bronchioles are infiltrated with inflammatory cells.
    Results in narrowing of respiratory passages and leads to hyperinflation of the alveoli.
35. etiologic agent
36. the clinical history, the child's age, the child's general health history, the physical examination, radiography, and the laboratory examination
37. Severe Acute Respiratory Syndrome (SARS)
38. *Mycobacterium tuberculosis*
39. chemotherapy
40. a. isoniazid (INH)
    b. rifampin (RMP)
    c. pyrazinamide (PZA)
41. avoid contact
42. false
43. they are naturally curious and tend to put everything in their mouths
44. choking, gagging, wheezing, or coughing
45. back blows, Heimlich maneuver
46. increased permeability
47. a. heat injury
    b. chemical injury
    c. systemic injury
48. Passive smoking

49. Chronic inflammatory disorder of the airways in which many cells may play a role. Inflammation causes airflow limitation or a narrowing of the airways. Obstruction is reversible either spontaneously or with treatment.
50. allergy (influences both the persistence and severity of the disease)
51. a. inflammation and edema of mucous membranes
    b. accumulation of tenacious secretions from mucous glands
    c. spasm of the smooth muscle of the bronchi and bronchioles, which decreases the caliber of the bronchioles
52. Air trapping; higher, higher
53. a. dyspnea or shortness of breath
    b. wheezing
    c. cough
54. prevent disability, physical, psychologic
55. Allergen
56. prevent and control asthma symptoms
57. corticosteroids
58. Bronchodilators
59. a. beta-adrenergics
    b. methylxanthines
60. Cromylyn sodium
61. peak expiratory flow rate
62. third-line
63. Leukotriene modifiers
64. It has been found that exercise is advantageous for children with asthma, provided their asthma is under control.
65. a. breathing exercises
    b. physical training
66. controversial
67. an asthma attack in which the child continues to display respiratory distress despite vigorous therapeutic measures
68. Beta$_2$-agonists and corticosteroids. If the child is not responding, epinephrine is also given.
69. metered-dose inhaler
70. a. Asthma is a very common disease that can be controlled.
    b. An asthmatic attack is easier to prevent than to treat.
    c. Persons with asthma are able to live full and active lives.
71. autosomal-recessive trait
72. mechanical obstruction caused by the increased viscosity of mucous gland secretions
73. meconium ileus
74. Because essential pancreatic enzymes are unable to reach the duodenum, digestion and absorption of nutrients are markedly impaired.
75. Pulmonary complications
76. large, frothy, and extremely foul-smelling
77. a. history of the disease in the family
    b. absence of pancreatic enzymes
    c. increase in electrolyte concentration of sweat
    d. chronic pulmonary involvement
78. sodium, chloride
79. a. to prevent or minimize pulmonary complications
    b. to ensure adequate nutrition for growth
    c. to encourage appropriate physical activity
    d. to promote a reasonable quality of life for the child and family
80. preventing and treating pulmonary infection
81. a. improving aeration
    b. removing mucopurlent secretions
    c. administering antimicrobial agents
82. Pulmozyme

83. a. with meals and snacks
    b. severity of insufficiency; response of the child to enzyme replacement; and philosophy of the physician
    c. normal growth and development and decrease of number of stools to one or two per day
84. well-balanced, high-protein, high-calorie, and supplemented with A, D, E, K vitamins; when high-fat foods consumed, must increase enzyme replacement
85. pulmonary involvement
86. a. (1) increased work of breathing but with gas exchange function near normal
        (2) inability to maintain normal blood gas tensions; development of hypoxemia and acidosis as result of CO_2 retention
    b. inability of the respiratory apparatus to maintain adequate oxygenation of the blood
    c. cessation of respiration
    d. cessation of breathing for more that 20 seconds or a shorter amount of time when associated with hypoxemia or bradycardia
87. hypoxemia
88. b
89. 1

Applying Critical Thinking to Nursing Practice

A.
  1. a. ineffective breathing pattern related to inflammatory process
     b. fear/anxiety related to difficulty breathing, unfamiliar procedures, and possibly environment (hospital)
     c. ineffective airway clearance related to mechanical obstruction, inflammation, increased secretions, pain
     d. risk for infection related to presence of infective organisms
     e. activity intolerance related to inflammatory process, imbalance between oxygen supply and demand
     f. pain related to inflammatory process, surgical incision
     g. altered family process related to illness and/or hospitalization of a child
B.
  1. Child would be irritable, crying, fussy, and pulling on her ears or rolling her head from side to side; she may have fever of as much as 104° F, anorexia, and signs of respiratory or pharyngeal infection.
  2. Complete course (10 or 14 days) of prescribed antibiotic.
C.
  1. Monitor respirations; auscultate lungs; observe color of skin and mucous membranes; observe for presence of hoarseness, stridor, and cough; monitor heart rate and regularity; observe for retractions; observe behavior.
  2. No. Prevent aspiration and decrease work of breathing.
  3. to decrease the edema of the respiratory tract
D.
  1. respiratory syncytial virus (RSV), parainfluenza; influenza, adenovirus
  2. *Mycoplasma pneumoniae*
  3. *Streptococcus*, *Staphylococcus*, *Pneumococcus*
  4. symptomatic
  5. symptomatic
  6. antimicrobial therapy directed at causative organism; pneumococcal polysaccharide vaccine
E.
  1. tuberculin skin test
  2. a. Two or more drugs are usually required.
     b. Drugs must be continued for a long time, so compliance is a concern.
  3. Yes, he can return to school if receiving chemotherapy. He does not need to be isolated because his disease is not contagious. Protect from stress. Get optimal nutrition and rest.
F.
  1. hacking, nonproductive cough; shortness of breath
  2. shortness of breath; productive cough; audible wheezing; deep, dark red color to the lips; cyanosis; restlessness and apprehension; sweating; use of accessory muscles; rapid respirations; upright position with hunched shoulders; speaking with short, panting broken phrases; wheezes throughout lung fields; prolonged expiration; and crackles.

3. a. relief of bronchospasm
   b. irritability, tremor, nervousness, and insomnia
4. Child sweats profusely, remains sitting upright, and refuses to lie down. A child who suddenly becomes agitated or suddenly becomes quiet may be seriously hypoxic.
5. a. Child will not experience an asthmatic episode.
   b. Child will exhibit improved ventilatory capacity.
   c. Child will maintain optimum health.
   d. Child will not develop complications.
   e. Child will engage in normal activities for age.
   f. Child and family will receive appropriate support and education regarding the disease and its management.
6. a. Child's respirations are unlabored and within normal limits.
   b. Child rests and sleeps comfortably.
   c. Child does not experience decreased oxygen saturations.
G.
1. a. ineffective airway clearance related to secretion of thick tenacious mucus
   b. impaired gas exchange related to airway obstruction
   c. ineffective breathing pattern related to tracheobronchial obstruction
   d. altered nutrition (less than body requirements) related to inability to digest nutrients
   e. altered growth and development related to inadequate digestion of nutrients
   f. risk for infection related to impaired body defenses, presence of mucus as medium for growth of organisms
   g. activity intolerance related to imbalance between oxygen supply and demand
   h. altered family process related to situational crisis
   i. impaired social interaction related to hospitalization, home confinement, fatigue
   j. anticipatory grieving related to perceived potential loss of child
2. Dennis manages secretions with minimum distress.
3. a. Bronchioles and bronchi are obstructed with abnormally thick mucus.
   b. Lack of trypsin, amylase, and lipase causes large amounts of undigested food, which are excreted.
   c. Because so little food is absorbed from the intestine, the child tries to compensate.
   d. Appetite can't compensate for fecal elimination and lack of absorption.
   e. Child is unable to absorb fat-soluble vitamins.
4. a. postural drainage technique
   b. breathing exercises
   c. aerosol therapy

Chapter 24

Review of Essential Concepts

1. the total output of fluid exceeds the total intake
2. c
3. true
4. isotonic, hypotonic, hypertonic
5. c
6. It is defined as a sudden increase in frequency and a change in consistency of stools.
7. false
8. d
9. fecal-oral
10. rotavirus
11. Giardia
12. true
13. decreased urine output; decreased weight; dry mucous membranes; poor skin turgor; sunken fontanel; and pale, cool, dry skin

14. a. meeting ongoing daily physiologic losses
    b. replacing previous deficits
    c. replacing ongoing abnormal losses
15. prevention
16. alteration in frequency, consistency, or ease of passing stool
17. Environmental change
18. ganglion cells
19. absence of propulsive movement
20. rectal biopsy
21. surgical correction
22. transfer of gastric contents into the esophagus
23. SIDS; left side, head of the bed
24. a. right lower quadrant abdominal pain
    b. fever
    c. rigid abdomen
    d. decreased or absent bowel sounds
    e. vomiting
    f. constipation or diarrhea
    g. anorexia
    h. tachycardia; rapid, shallow breathing
    i. pallor
    j. lethargy
    k. irritability
    l. stooped posture
25. McBurney's point, anterior superior iliac crest and the umbilicus
26. false
27. a remnant of the fetal-omphalo-mesenteric duct that connects the yolk sac with the primitive midgut during fetal life; normally closes in the 7th to 8th week of gestation
28. the diverticulum contains gastric mucosa, which produces hydrochloric acid, which irritates the bowel and erodes the intestinal surface, causing ulceration and perforation
29. history; physical examination; specialized radiographic studies
30. surgical removal
31. ulcerative colitis
32. a. corticosteroids
    b. aminosalicylates
    c. sulfasalazine
    d. immunomodulatory therapies (azathioprine, 6MP, etc.)
    e. biologic therapies (Remicade, Methotrexate, etc.)
    f. variety of antibiotics
33. ulcerative colitis
34. epigastric pain or vague abdominal pain; nighttime waking; hematemesis; melena and anemia
35. a. to relieve discomfort
    b. to promote healing
    c. to prevent complications
    d. to prevent recurrence
36. a. hepatitis A virus (HAV)
    b. hepatitis B virus (HBV)
    c. hepatitis C virus (HCV)
    d. hepatitis D virus (HDV)
    e. hepatitis E virus (HEV)
    f. hepatitis G virus (HGV)
37. a. oral, fecal
    b. parenteral
    c. usually rapid acute
    d. more insidious

38. a. history
    b. physical examination
    c. serologic markers in A, B, C
    d. elevated serum aspartate and alanine aminotransferase levels
39. a. true
    b. true
    c. false
    d. true
    e. true
40. a. frequent assessment of liver status with physical examination and liver function tests
    b. management of specific complications
41. hepatic portoenterostomy (Kasai procedure)
42. defective speech
43. feeding
44. a. excessive salivation and drooling
    b. coughing, choking, cyanosis
    c. apnea
    d. increased respiratory distress following feeding
    e. abdominal distention
45. coughing, choking, cyanosis
46. protrusion of a portion of an organ or organs through an abnormal opening
47. incarcerated
48. projectile
49. pyloromyotomy
50. occurs when a proximal segment of the bowel telescopes into a more distal portion, pulling the mesentery with it
51. barium enema
52. malrotation; volvulus
53. Malabsorption syndrome
54. a. digestive defects
    b. absorptive defects
    c. anatomic defects
55. a. impaired fat absorption
    b. impaired absorption of nutrients
    c. behavioral changes
    d. celiac crisis
56. celiac crisis
57. a. to preserve as much length of bowel as possible during surgery
    b. to maintain the child's nutritional status and growth and development while intestinal adaptation occurs
    c. to stimulate the intestinal adaptation with enteral feeding
    d. to minimize complications related to the disease process and therapy

Applying Critical Thinking to Nursing Practice

A.
 1. fluid volume deficit related to excessive GI losses in stool or emesis
 2. c
 3. Child has no evidence of skin breakdown.
B.
 1. a. accurate history of bowel habits
    b. diet and events that may be associated with the onset of constipation
    c. drugs or other substances that the child may be taking
    d. consistency, color, frequency, and other characteristics of the stool

C.
1. a. creation of temporary colostomy
   b. surgical correction when child weighs 9 kg
   c. closure of colostomy (may be done simultaneously with second stage)
D.
1. a. This therapy decreases the number of episodes of vomiting and increases the caloric density of the formula.
   b. Add 1 teaspoon to 1 tablespoon of rice cereal (as directed by physician) to each ounce of formula. Make hole in nipple larger to facilitate feeding.
2. a. identifying children with symptoms of GER
   b. educating parents regarding home care including feeding, positioning, and medications when indicated
   c. providing care if child requires surgical repair
E.
1. degree of change in his behavior
2. Patient will experience minimized risk for spread of infection.
3. a. listen for return of bowel sounds
   b. observe for passage of stool
4. Child does not exhibit signs of discomfort; abdomen remains soft and nondistended; child does not vomit.
F.
1. Inflammation is limited to the colon and rectum. Inflammation affects the mucosa and submucosa and involves continuous segments with varying degrees of ulceration, bleeding, and edema.
2. affects the terminal ileum and involves all layers of bowel wall (transmural) in a discontinuous fashion
3. common
4. uncommon
5. often severe
6. moderate to absent
7. less frequent
8. common
9. mild or moderate
10. may be severe
11. moderate
12. may be severe
13. usually mild
14. may be severe
G.
1. a. severity of hepatitis
   b. medical management
   c. factors influencing control and transmission of the disease
2. a well-balanced diet and a realistic schedule of rest and activity adjusted to the child's condition
H.
1. The feeding process is often time-consuming and very difficult. Clefts of the lip or palate reduce the infant's ability to suck, which interferes with compression of the areola and usually renders both breast- and bottle-feeding difficult.
2. a. Infant will experience no trauma to operative site.
   b. Infant will exhibit no evidence of aspiration.
   c. Infant will consume adequate nourishment.
   d. Infant will experience optimum comfort level.
   e. Infant and family will receive adequate support.
3. Operative site remains undamaged.
I.
1. a. Give small frequent feedings of clear liquids.
   b. Bubble before and frequently during feedings.
   c. Position child with head elevated.
2. Vomiting may continue contributing to lost fluids and electrolytes.
   Monitoring of oral intake and IV intake along with output will guard against dehydration.

J.
1. a. (1) Explain diagnosis; (2) encourage parents to room-in; (3) explain procedures and equipment; (4) support parents through this sudden emergency.
   b. (1) Explain and demonstrate why this procedure is being performed; (2) assure the parents that you will accompany Jared to x-ray and support the child through the procedure.
K.
1. foods containing wheat, rye, barley, and oats
2. corn, rice

Chapter 25

Review of Essential Concepts

1. a
2. foramen ovale, ductus arteriosus
3. False
4. acyanotic, cyanotic
5. left, right
6. right, left
7. a. increased pulmonary blood flow
   b. decreased pulmonary blood flow
   c. obstruction to blood flow from ventricles
   d. mixed blood flow in which saturated and desaturated blood mix within the heart or great arteries
8. a. 1
   b. 2
   c. 2
   d. 1
   e. 1
   f. 1
   g. 2
9. a. 1
   b. 4
   c. 5
   d. 3
   e. 6
10. a. 1
    b. 1
    c. 2
    d. 2
    e. 2
    f. 2
11. a. 1
    b. 3
    c. 5
    d. 6
12. the inability of the heart to pump an adequate amount of blood to the systemic circulation at normal filling pressures to meet the body's metabolic demands
13. increased blood volume, pressure
14. a. right-sided failure
    b. left-sided failure
15. a. impaired myocardial function
    b. pulmonary congestion
    c. systemic venous congestion

16. tachycardia
17. tachypnea, dyspnea, retractions, flaring nares, exercise intolerance, orthopnea, cough, hoarseness, cyanosis, wheezing, grunting
18. weight gain, hepatomegaly, peripheral edema, ascites, and neck vein distention
19. a. Improve cardiac function.
    b. Remove accumulated fluid and sodium.
    c. Decrease cardiac demands.
    d. Improve tissue oxygenation and decrease oxygen consumption.
20. nausea, vomiting, anorexia, bradycardia, dysrhythmias
21. a. false
    b. true
    c. false
    d. true
    e. false
    f. true
    g. true
22. a. Allow a period of grief.
    b. Accept initial shock and disbelief.
    c. Foster parent-child attachment.
    d. Assess and assist with the effect of the child's illness on the whole family.
    e. Assist the family with maintaining discipline.
    f. Educate parents on how to avoid being overprotective of the child.
    g. Educate the family on the child's need for social development.
    h. Introduce parents to other families who have a similarly affected child.
23. *Streptococcus viridans*
24. cardiac valves
25. group A streptococcal
26. Jones, streptococcal; ASO
27. a. contain low concentrations of triglycerides, high levels of cholesterol, and moderate levels of protein
    b. contain very low concentrations of triglycerides, relatively little cholesterol, and high levels of protein
28. children and adolescents who have a family history of premature cardiovascular disease or at least one parent with blood cholesterol of 240 mg/dL or higher
29. a. bradydysrhythmias—abnormally slow rate
    b. tachydysrhythmias—abnormally rapid rate
    c. conduction disturbances—irregular heart rate
30. pacemaker
31. Cardiomyopathy
32. cardiomyopathy, end-stage congenital heart disease
33. blood pressure
34. Kawasaki disease, cardiovascular
35. temperature
36. aspirin, gamma globulin
37. a. hypotension
    b. tissue hypoxia
    c. metabolic acidosis
38. a. hypovolemic shock
    b. distributive shock
    c. cardiogenic shock
39. a. compensated
    b. uncompensated
    c. irreversible or terminal shock
40. a. ventilation
    b. fluid administration
    c. improvement of the pumping action of the heart

41. the interaction of an allergen and a patient who is hypersensitive
42. flushing; urticaria; angioedema—noticed in eyelids, lips, tongue, hands, feet, and genitalia

Applying Critical Thinking to Nursing Practice

A.
1. height; weight; history of allergic reactions; signs and symptoms of infection; baseline oxygen saturation; and locate and mark pedal pulses
2. a. detects abnormalities in rate and rhythm
   b. detects cardiac hemorrhage from perforation or bleeding at the site of the initial catheterization
   c. detects vessel obstruction
   d. detects possible arterial obstruction

B.
1. a. maternal health history; pregnancy; birth history; maternal rubella; poor nutrition; maternal insulin-dependent diabetes; maternal age over 40 years; maternal alcoholism; maternal chronic health problems; drug use by mother; exposure to rubella
   b. increased risk for congenital heart disease in a child who (1) has a sibling with a heart defect; (2) has a parent with congenital heart disease; (3) has a chromosomal aberration, especially Down syndrome; or (4) is born with other noncardiac congenital anomalies
2. a loud, harsh, pansystolic murmur
3. Feed on 3-hour schedule; feed small amounts that are calorie-dense; provide soft, large-hole preemie nipple and hold in semi-upright position. Allow to rest frequently. May need to encourage sucking.

C.
1. a. improves cardiac functioning by such beneficial effects as increased cardiac output, decreased heart size, decreased venous pressure, and relief of edema
   b. removes accumulated fluid and sodium
2. a. Count the apical pulse for 1 full minute before administering digitalis, and withhold dose if pulse is lower than either 90–110 in infants or 70 in older children.
   b. Calculate dosage accurately; check with another nurse.
   c. Use correct preparation of digitalis (use digoxin).
   d. Monitor serum potassium levels.
3. Low potassium increases the cardiac effects of digitalis.
4. nausea, vomiting, anorexia, bradycardia, dysrhythmias
5. a. Any two of the following are acceptable:
   Place in an inclined posture of 30-45 degrees.
   Avoid any constricting clothing or restraints around abdomen and chest.
   Administer humidified oxygen as prescribed.
   Assess respiratory rate, ease of respiration, color, and oxygen saturation as measured by oximetry.
   b. Any two of the following are acceptable:
   Maintain a neutral thermal environment.
   Keep infant warm—place newborn in incubator or under warmer.
   Treat fever promptly.
   Feed small volumes at frequent intervals; implement gavage feeding if infant becomes fatigued before taking adequate amount.
   Time nursing activities to disturb child as little as possible.
   Implement measures to reduce anxiety; respond promptly to crying or distress.
   c. Any two of the following are acceptable:
   Employ a flexible feeding schedule.
   Handle the child gently; hold and comfort the infant; employ comfort measures found effective for the individual child.
   Encourage the family to provide comfort and solace.
   Explain equipment and procedures to the child.

    d. Any two of the following are acceptable:
        Administer diuretics as ordered.
        Carefully monitor intake and output; monitor body weight.
        Assess for evidence of increased or decreased edema; maintain fluid restriction.
        Provide skin care for children with edema; change position frequently; use alternating pressure mattress.
D.
  1. a. fluid volume deficit related to increased body temperature
      b. sensory-perceptual alterations (visual) related to inflammation of the eyes
      c. altered nutrition, less than body requirements, related to inadequate intake
      d. potential impaired skin integrity related to irritation of edematous tissue and denuded skin
      e. pain related to itchy rash
      f. pain related to swelling in cervical region
  2. a. Administer aspirin, teach the family signs of aspirin toxicity, monitor the temperature frequently, promote rest.
      b. Encourage fluids, keep accurate intake and output records, take and record daily weight, monitor temperature status, assess skin turgor, monitor urine specific gravity.
      c. Administer aspirin as ordered, observe for signs of myocarditis and congestive heart failure, monitor vital signs frequently, observe for behavioral changes, teach parents the need for close follow-up care.
E.
  1. a. Family and child will adjust to the diagnosis.
      b. Family will be knowledgeable regarding symptoms of the disease and the management.
      c. Family will cope with effects of the disorder.
      d. Child and family will be prepared for surgical repair of defect.
      e. Child undergoing cardiac surgery will receive appropriate care.
      f. Family will receive adequate emotional support.
      g. Family will be prepared for home care.
  2. Discuss with parents their fears and concerns regarding the child's cardiac defects and physical symptoms. Encourage the family to participate in the child's care. Encourage the family to include others in the child's care to prevent exhaustion. Assist the family in determining appropriate physical activity.
  3. Rose can have patient-controlled intravenous analgesia after surgery, which the parents can control. Epidural medication is another option to control pain.
      The nurse would also teach Rose's parents a number of nonpharmacologic measures to decrease pain.

Chapter 26

Review of Essential Concepts

  1. a. red blood cell (RBC)
      b. hemoglobin (Hgb)
      c. hematocrit (Hct)
      d. RBC indices
      e. RBC volume distribution
      f. reticulocyte count
      g. white blood cell (WBC)
      h. differential WBC count
      i. absolute neutrophil count
      j. platelet count
      k. stained peripheral blood smear
  2. shift to the left
  3. reduction of red blood cell count
  4. a. etiology and physiology—manifested by erythrocyte and/or hemoglobin depletion
      b. morphology—the characteristic changes in red cell size, shape, and/or color
  5. a decrease in the oxygen-carrying capacity of the blood and a resulting reduction in amount of oxygen available to the cells

6. a. 4
   b. 6
   c. 8
   d. 7
   e. 5
   f. 3
   g. 2
   h. 1

7. a. average or mean volume of a single RBC
   b. mean quantity of hemoglobin in a single RBC
   c. mean concentration of hemoglobin in a single RBC
   d. number of RBC/mm^3 of blood
   e. amount of Hgb/dL of whole blood
   f. percentage or volume of packed RBC to whole blood
   g. percentage of reticulocytes to RBCs
   h. number of WBC/mm^3 of blood
   i. inspection and quantification of WBC types present in peripheral blood
   j. number of platelets in blood

8. reverse, deficiency

9. a. Prepare the child and family for laboratory tests.
   b. Decrease the tissue oxygen needs of the child.
   c. Prevent complications of anemia.

10. tachycardia, palpitations, tachypnea, dyspnea, shortness of breath, hyperpnea, breathlessness, dizziness, light-headedness, diaphoresis, change in skin color, fatigue

11. Iron

12. Children become anemic because they drink milk, a poor source of iron, almost to the exclusion of solid foods.

13. a. iron-fortified commercial formula
    b. iron-fortified infant cereal

14. vomiting, staining of teeth

15. prevention of nutritional anemia through education of family

16. tarry green color

17. a. heterozygous persons who have both normal HbA and abnormal HbS
    b. homozygous persons who have predominantly HbS and have sickle cell anemia

18. sickle-shaped

19. a. obstruction caused by sickled RBCs
    b. increased RBC destruction

20. a. stasis with enlargement
    b. infarction with ischemia and destruction
    c. replacement with fibrous tissue (scarring)

21. a. vasoocclusive crisis
    b. sequestration crisis
    c. aplastic crisis
    d. hyperhemolytic crisis

22. Sickledex

23. a. bed rest to minimize energy expenditure and oxygen use
    b. hydration through oral and IV therapy
    c. electrolyte replacement
    d. analgesics for severe pain from vasoocclusion
    e. blood replacement to treat anemia and reduce viscosity of sickled blood
    f. antibiotics to treat any existing infection

24. No

25. can depress bone marrow activity and further aggravate the anemia

26. Meperidine

27. Cooley anemia, compatible

28. red blood cells, anemia; hemosiderosis
29. Deferoxamine (Desferal)
30. a. primary (congenital)
    b. secondary (acquired)
31. immunosuppressive therapy, bone marrow transplant
32. a group of bleeding disorders in which there is a deficiency of one of the factors necessary for coagulation of blood
33. Classic hemophilia
    a. factor VIII
    b. factor IX
34. X-linked recessive disorder
35. joint space
36. missing clotting factor
37. Factor VIII concentrate, vasopressin (DDAVP)
38. should not, inhibit
39. HIV
40. a. thrombocytopenia, excessive destruction of platelets
    b. purpura (a discoloration caused by petechiae beneath the skin)
41. 20,000 mm^3; supportive
42. false
43. sitting up and leaning forward
44. a. acute lymphoid leukemia (ALL)
    b. acute myelogenous leukemia (AML)
45. a. a low leukocyte count but a greatly increased count of immature cells or "blasts"
    b. cellular destruction in the bone marrow by infiltration and subsequent competition for metabolic elements
46. a. anemia
    b. infection
    c. bleeding tendencies
    d. bone weakness and invasion of periosteum
47. pallor, fatigue, fever, hemorrhage, tendency toward bone fractures, and pain
48. bone marrow aspiration or biopsy
49. a. induction therapy
    b. CNS prophylactic therapy
    c. intensification or consolidation therapy
    d. maintenance therapy
50. central nervous system
51. a. corticosteroids; vincristine; and L-asparaginase, with or without doxorubicin, daunomycin, and cytosine arabinoside
    b. methotrexate, cytarabine, hydrocortisone
    c. L-asparaginase, methotrexate, cytarabine, vincristine, mercaptopurine
    d. mercaptopurine, methotrexate
52. the initial white blood count; the child's age at diagnosis; the histologic type of the cell involved; sex; karyotype analysis
53. a. Hodgkin disease originates in the lymphoid system and primarily involves the lymph nodes. It predictably metastasizes to non-nodal or extralymphatic sites, especially the spleen, liver, bone marrow, and lungs.
    b. Non-Hodgkin lymphoma in children is strikingly different from Hodgkin disease. The disease is usually diffuse, rather than nodular; the cell type is either undifferentiated or poorly differentiated; dissemination occurs early, more often than in Hodgkin disease, and rapidly; mediastinal involvement and invasion of meninges are common.
54. radiation, chemotherapy
55. intimate sexual contact; exposure to blood or body fluids; passed from mother to fetus

56. a. perinatal transmission (in utero, delivery, breast-feeding)
    b. receiving tainted blood products through transfusion
    c. adolescents infected during sexual activity or children during sexual abuse
57. preventing transmission of the virus
58. a. HIV
    b. no cure; primarily slowing growth of virus; prevention and management of the opportunistic infections; providing nutritional support and symptomatic treatment; use of antiviral drugs; prophylaxis for *Pneumocystis carinii* pneumonia with trimethoprim sulfamethoxazole (TMP/SMZ); prophylaxis for disseminated *Mycobacterium* avium-intracellulare complex (MAC), candidiasis, and herpes simplex; immunizations; and nutritional management
    c. changing from fatal to chronic disease
59. a defect characterized by absence of both humoral and cell-mediated immunity
60. hematopoietic stem cell transplant (HSCT)
61. a. thrombocytopenia
    b. eczema
    c. immunodeficiency of selective functions of B- and T-lymphocytes
62. a. hemolytic reactions
    b. febrile reactions
    c. allergic reactions
    d. circulatory overload
    e. air emboli
    f. hypothermia
    g. electrolyte disturbances
63. a. allogenic
    b. umbilical cord blood stem cell
    c. autologous
    d. peripheral stem cell
64. removal of blood from an individual; the separation of the blood into its components and the retention of one or more of these components; and the remainder of blood reinfused into the individual

Applying Critical Thinking to Nursing Practice

A.
1. a. explaining the significance of each test
   b. encouraging parents or another supportive person to be with the child during the procedure
   c. allowing the child to play with the equipment on a doll and/or participate in the actual procedure
2. a. anxiety/fear related to diagnostic procedures/transfusion
   b. activity intolerance related to generalized weakness, diminished oxygen delivery to tissues
   c. altered nutrition (less than body requirements) related to reported inadequate iron intake; knowledge deficit regarding iron-rich foods

B.
1. a. pain related to tissue ischemia
   b. altered tissue perfusion related to impaired arterial blood flow
2. Analyze the current drug dosage and suggest an increase to prevent rather than treat pain. Add psychologic support to counter depression, anxiety, and fear. Administer medication "around the clock" or PCA.
3. Few, if any, children who receive opioids for severe pain become behaviorally addicted to the drug. When the pain is gone, need for the drug is gone. Addiction is rare.

C.
1. a. rest
   b. ice
   c. compression
   d. elevation
2. use of a water irrigating device; soft toothbrush; softening toothbrush in warm water; use of a sponge-tipped disposable toothbrush

D.
1. a. Patient will exhibit no evidence of bleeding.
    b. Patient will exhibit no evidence of hemorrhagic cystitis.
    c. Patient will experience minimal effects of anemia.
2. a. Provide meticulous skin care, especially in mouth and perianal regions.
    b. Change position frequently.
    c. Encourage adequate calorie-protein intake.
3. a. because they are prone to ulceration
    b. to stimulate circulation and relieve pressure
    c. to prevent negative nitrogen balance
E.
1. a. Implement and carry out standard precautions.
    b. Instruct others in appropriate precautions; clarify any misconceptions about communicability of virus.
    c. Teach affected children protective methods.
    d. Endeavor to keep infants and small children from placing hands and objects in contaminated areas.
    e. Place restrictions on behaviors and contacts for affected children who bite or who do not have control of bodily secretions.
    f. Assess the home situation and implement protective measures as feasible in individual circumstances.
2. a. risk for infection related to impaired body defenses, presence of infective organisms
    b. altered nutrition (less than body requirements) related to recurrent illness, diarrheal losses, loss of appetite, oral candidiasis
    c. impaired social interaction related to physical limitations, hospitalizations, social stigma toward HIV infection
    d. altered sexuality patterns related to risk for disease transmission
    e. chronic pain related to disease process
    f. interrupted family processes related to having a child with a dreaded and life-threatening disease
    g. anticipatory grief related to having a child with a potentially fatal illness

Chapter 27

Review of Essential Concepts

1. urinalysis
2. a. 4
    b. 2
    c. 1
    d. 5
    e. 3
3. urinary stasis
4. false
5. a. incontinence if toilet-trained
    b. strong-smelling urine
    c. frequency and/or urgency
6. a. Eliminate current infection.
    b. Identify contributing factors to reduce the risk for recurrence.
    c. Prevent systemic spread of the infection.
    d. Preserve renal function.
7. refers to the abnormal retrograde flow of bladder urine into the ureters
8. a. congenital or acquired
    b. unilateral or bilateral
    c. complete or incomplete
    d. acute or chronic

9. a. dilation of the renal pelvis due to urine collection
   b. fluid in scrotum
   c. meatal opening located on dorsal surface of penis
   d. narrowing or stenosis of preputial opening of foreskin
   e. failure of one or both testes to descend normally through inguinal canal
10. b
11. c
12. Corticosteroids
13. a
14. a. 2
    b. 2
    c. 1
    d. 2
    e. 1
15. a. history of a sore throat and/or skin infection
    b. urine analysis
    c. ASO titer
    d. elevated antihyaluronidase (AHase) and antideoxyribonuclease B (ADNase-B) titers and streptozyme levels
    e. decreased serum complement levels
    f. chest x-ray
16. false
17. true
18. proximal tubules; glomeruli
19. true
20. Hemolytic uremic syndrome
21. the lining of the small glomerular arterioles
22. a. vomiting
    b. irritability
    c. lethargy
    d. pallor
    e. hemorrhagic manifestations
    f. anuria or oliguria
    g. central nervous system involvement
    h. signs of acute heart failure
23. the damage to the red blood cells in the arterioles and the subsequent hemolysis; the damaged cells are removed by the spleen
24. Wilms tumor
25. surgery, chemotherapy, radiation
26. Chemotherapy
27. c
28. oliguria
29. a. treatment of the underlying cause
    b. management of the complications of renal failure
    c. provision of supportive therapy
30. hyperkalemia, hypertension
31. true
32. the process of separating colloids and crystalline substances in solution by the difference in their rate of diffusion through a semipermeable membrane
33. a. peritoneal dialysis
    b. hemodialysis
    c. hemofiltration
34. peritoneal dialysis
35. renal transplantation

Applying Critical Thinking to Nursing Practice

A.
1. a. fever
   b. voiding large amounts
   c. poor feeding
2. The incidence of UTI in males is greater in infancy. This is usually the result of some sort of obstruction that results in urinary stasis. Also, the presence of a large or greater than normal output is suggestive of obstructive uropathy.
3. prevention
4. a. Collect a specimen.
   b. Prepare Barry's parents for the diagnostic procedure.
   c. Administer antimicrobials as ordered.
   d. Monitor vital signs.
   e. Increase fluid intake.
   f. Monitor urine output.
   g. Teach Barry's parents how to perform his home care.
   h. Teach Barry's parents how to prevent recurrences.

B.
1. fluid volume excess related to fluid accumulation in tissues and third spaces
2. Child will exhibit no evidence of infection.
3. The presence of edema may predispose the child to skin breakdown and may make routine care more difficult.
4. Put a cottonball in the diaper especially at night. The nurse can squeeze urine from the cottonball with ease for specimen collection.

C.
1. The nurse should have instructed Tina's mother to continue the antibiotics for the total prescribed time, even if Tina felt better.
2. a. Monitor fluid and electrolyte balance.
   b. Weigh the child daily.
   c. Measure intake and output.
   d. Measure specific gravity of urine.
   e. Observe for signs of dehydration and overload.
   f. Monitor vital signs.
3. The parents will demonstrate testing of urine and vital signs correctly. They will verbalize the instructions regarding other measures with accuracy.

D.
1. vomiting, irritability, lethargy, pallor, hemorrhagic manifestations, oliguria or anuria, central nervous system manifestations, signs of heart failure
2. a. the disease, its implications, and the therapeutic plan
   b. the possible psychologic effects of the disease and its treatment
   c. the technical aspects of the procedure
3. patient will consume appropriate diet
4. will maintain near-normal electrolyte levels
5. Child and family demonstrate ability to cope with stresses of illness.

E.
1. a. Keep explanations simple, and repeat them often.
   b. Focus on the child's actual experiences.
2. a. monitoring bowel movements
   b. auscultating for bowel sounds
   c. monitoring for abdominal distention or vomiting
   c. monitoring for pain

Chapter 28

Review of Essential Concepts

1. a. observing spontaneous and elicited reflex responses
   b. eliciting progressively more sophisticated communicative and adaptive behaviors
   c. observing for the presence of a primitive reflex beyond the time it would normally disappear
   d. obtaining the pregnancy and delivery history
2. a. family history
   b. health history
   c. physical evaluation of infants
3. a. tense, bulging fontanel; separated cranial sutures; Macewen sign; irritability; high-pitched cry; increased occipital frontal circumference; distended scalp veins; change in feeding patterns; cries when disturbed; "setting sun" sign
   b. headache; nausea; vomiting; diplopia; seizures; irritability; drowsiness; decline in school performance; diminished physical activity and motor performance; increased sleeping; memory loss; inability to follow commands; lethargy and drowsiness
4. bradycardia; lowered level of consciousness; decreased motor response to command; decreased sensory response to painful stimuli; alterations in pupil size and reactivity; sometimes decerebrate or decorticate posturing; Cheyne-Stokes respiration; papilledema; coma
5. a. alertness: an aroused or waking state that includes the ability to respond to stimuli
   b. cognitive power: the ability to process stimuli and produce verbal and motor responses
6. the child's responses to the environment
7. a. 3
   b. 8
   c. 1
   d. 5
   e. 2
   f. 7
   g. 6
   h. 4
8. a. eye opening
   b. verbal response
   c. motor response
9. establish an accurate, objective baseline of neurologic function
10. vital signs, skin, eyes, motor function, posturing, and reflexes
11. emergency
12. a. adduction of arms at the shoulders, flexion of arms on the chest with the wrist flexed and the hands fisted, and extension and adduction of the lower extremities
   b. rigid extension and pronation of arms and legs
13. a. lumbar puncture
   b. subdural tap
   c. electroencephalogram (EEG)
   d. video EEG
   e. computerized tomography (CT)
   f. nuclear brain scan
   g. transillumination
   h. echoencephalography
   i. radiography
   j. magnetic resonance imaging (MRI)
   k. positron emission transaxial tomography (PETT) or positron emission tomography (PET)
   l. real-time ultrasonography (RTUS)
   m. digital substraction angiography (DSA)
14. patent airway

15. a. intraventricular catheter with fibroscopic sensors attached to a monitoring system
     b. subarachnoid bolt
     c. epidural sensor
     d. anterior fontanel pressure monitor
16. a. bruising of the brain at point of impact
     b. bruising of brain at a distance as the brain collides with the unyielding surface of the skull, far removed from point of impact
17. a. concussion: a transient and reversible neuronal dysfunction with instantaneous loss of awareness and responsiveness for minutes or hours
     b. contusion and laceration: visible bruising and tearing of cerebral tissue
     c. fracture: a break in the skull that is linear, depressed, comminuted basilar, open or diastatic
18. hemorrhage; infection; edema; herniation through the tentorium
19. Accumulation of blood between the skull and cerebral surfaces is dangerous because it can compress the underlying brain and produce effects that can be rapidly fatal or insidiously progressive.
20. hematoma
21. dura, cerebrum, cortical veins
22. cerebral
23. Intracranial pressure exceeds arterial pressure, and fatal anoxia ensues, and/or the pressure causes herniation of a portion of the brain over the edge of the tentorium, compressing the brain stem and occluding the posterior cerebral arteries.
24. computed tomography
25. assessment of the child's LOC and ICP
26. the length of submersion, the physiologic response of the victim, and the development and degree of immersion hypothermia
27. a. hypoxia and asphyxiation
     b. aspiration
     c. hypothermia
28. prevented
29. infratentorial; supratentorial
30. because their sutures are still open and an increase in the size of the head is not readily detected
31. magnetic resonance imaging (MRI)
32. removal
33. infectious process
34. cerebral edema
35. adrenal gland, retroperitoneal sympathetic chain
36. primary site, areas of metastasis
37. catecholamines
38. surgery, radiotherapy, chemotherapy
39. regression
40. a. meninges (meningitis)
     b. brain (encephalitis)
     c. spinal cord (myelitis)
41. Hib
42. a. *Streptococcus pneumoniae*
     b. *Neisseria meningitidis (Meningococcus)*
43. Meningococcal meningitis is readily transmitted by droplet infection from nasopharyngeal secretions.
44. a. false
     b. false
     c. false
45. symptomatic
46. a. direct invasion of the central nervous system by a virus
     b. postinfectious involvement of the central nervous system after a viral disease
47. influenza, varicella
48. aspirin
49. unexplained neurodevelopmental regression and focal seizures

50. a. the inactivated rabies vaccines
    b. the globulins, which contain preformed antibodies
51. a spontaneous electric discharge is initiated by a group of hyperexcitable cells referred to as the epileptogenic focus. When neuronal excitation from the epileptogenic focus spreads to the brain stem, a generalized seizure develops.
52. partial seizures and generalized seizures
53. a period of altered behavior for which the individual is amnesic and during which he or she is unable to respond to the environment. There is no loss of consciousness during the attack, only impaired consciousness. Drowsiness or sleep follow the seizure. Confusion and amnesia are prolonged. Complex sensory phenomena occur as well as strong feelings of fear and anxiety; small children emit a cry or attempt to run for help.
54. electroencephalogram (EEG)
55. a. Control the seizures or reduce their frequency.
    b. Discover and correct the cause of seizures when possible.
    c. Help the child who has recurrent seizures to live as normal a life as possible.
56. The action of anticonvulsive drugs is to raise the threshold of excitability and prevent seizures.
57. The drugs are monitored by taking frequent serum drug levels.
58. The drug should be reduced gradually over 1 to 2 weeks.
59. grand mal, generalized
60. petit mal, absence
61. a continuous seizure that lasts more than 30 minutes or as serial seizures from which the child does not regain a premorbid level of consciousness
62. siderails raised when child is sleeping; siderails padded; waterproof mattress/pad on bed/crib; appropriate precautions during potentially hazardous activities; have child carry or wear medical identification; alert other caregivers to need for any special precautions; identify and avoid triggering factors whenever possible
63. transient disorders of children that occur in association with a fever
64. normal
65. Hydrocephalus
66. a. impaired absorption of CSF within the subarachnoid space (communicating)
    b. obstruction to the flow of CSF within the ventricles (noncommunicating)
67. a. abnormally rapid head growth
    b. bulging fontanels
    c. dilated scalp veins
    d. separated sutures
    e. Macewen sign on percussion
    f. thinning of skull bones
    g. frontal enlargement or "bossing"
    h. depressed eyes—"setting sun" sign
    i. sluggish pupils with unequal response to light
68. true
69. CAT scan, MRI
70. ventriculoperitoneal (VP)

Applying Critical Thinking to Nursing Practice

A.
1. alteration in neurologic status related to increased intracranial pressure
2. lethargy

B.
1. Any three of the following are acceptable:
   Child will maintain respiratory integrity.
   Child will not experience increasing ICP.
   Child will have basic needs met.
   Child will not experience complications of immobility.
   Family will receive adequate support and education.

2. vital signs, pupillary reactions, level of consciousness
3. a. elevating head of bed 15 to 30 degrees
   b. avoiding positions or activities that increase ICP
   c. preventing constipation
   d. minimizing emotional stress and crying
   e. preventing or relieving pain
   f. scheduling disturbing procedures to take advantage of therapies that reduce ICP
   g. monitoring ICP monitoring device
4. to prevent tissue breakdown and pressure necrosis
5. Child exhibits no signs of sustained increased ICP.

C.
1. vital signs, neurologic signs, and level of consciousness
2. Assure parents that everything possible is being done to treat the child; repeat the message often. It is important for parents to know they are not alone.

D.
1. Clinical manifestations include fever, poor feeding, vomiting, marked irritability, seizures, a high-pitched cry, and a bulging fontanel. Nuchal rigidity may or may not be present. Brudzinski and Kernig signs are not usually used in making the diagnosis, since they are difficult to evaluate in children in this age group.
2. a. isolation precautions
   b. environmental stimuli kept at minimum
   c. position on side or with HOB elevated
   d. institute seizure precautions
   e. observe vital signs, neurologic signs, LOC, intake and output frequently
   f. measure head circumference daily
   g. maintain IV antimicrobial therapy
   h. support family

E.
1. a. description of child's behavior before and during a seizure
   b. the age of onset of first seizure
   c. the usual time at which the seizure occurs
   d. any factors that may have precipitated the seizure
   e. any sensory phenomena that the child can describe
   f. duration and progression of the seizure
   g. postictal feelings and behavior
2. a. Do not attempt to restrain child or use force.
   b. Remove objects in bed.
   c. Place pillow or folded blanket under child's head.
   d. Do not force object between clenched teeth.
   e. Protect her from injury on siderails.
   f. Allow seizures to end without interference.
3. a. Help the family to establish time of administration of medication to coincide with the family routine.
   b. The tablet form of the drug is the preferred form; crush and administer in syrup or jelly.
   c. Emphasize that the medication must be continued for as long as required.
   d. Explain the need for adequate vitamin D and folic acid.
   e. Do not take with milk.
   f. Teach what side effects may occur.
   g. Explain why periodic blood studies are necessary.
   h. Explain the degree to which activities are restricted.

F.
1. a. positioning on the unoperated side to prevent pressure on the shunt valve
   b. keeping flat to prevent too rapid reduction of intracranial fluid
   c. managing pain with Tylenol, Tylenol with codeine, or opioids
   d. monitoring neurologic status
   e. monitoring vital signs
   f. monitoring abdominal girth

g. monitoring hydration status
h. monitoring for infection of operative site
i. inspecting incision site for leakage
j. meticulous skin care
2. Family discusses their feelings and concerns regarding the child's condition.

Chapter 29

Review of Essential Concepts

1. hypophysis, master gland
2. Idiopathic factors
3. short stature
4. growth hormone
5. a. surgical removal or irradiation of tumor
   b. replacement of growth hormone
6. overgrowth of long bones; overgrowth in transverse direction, acromegaly
7. increasing intracranial pressure
8. early identification of children with inappropriate growth rates
9. diabetes insipidus, diuresis
10. polyuria, polydipsia
11. vasopressin; desmopressin acetate
12. syndrome of inappropriate secretion of antidiuretic hormone
13. fluid retention and hypotonicity
14. thyroid
15. to regulate the basal metabolic rate
16. thyroid hormone
17. an enlargement or hypertrophy of the thyroid gland; iodine
18. thyroid gland
19. acute onset; severe irritability and restlessness; vomiting; diarrhea; hyperthermia; hypertension; severe tachycardia; prostration; may progress to delirium, coma, death
20. hypoparathyroidism
21. calcium, phosphate
22. Hyperparathyroidism
23. a. 1
    b. 2
    c. 2
    d. 1
    e. 1
24. a. 1
    b. 2
25. iatrogenic Cushing syndrome
26. moon
27. sexual
28. genotype
29. adrenogenital hyperplasia
30. dominant
31. increased production of catecholamines
32. a. glucagon: stimulates liver to release stored glucose
    b. insulin: facilitates entrance of glucose into the cells for metabolism
    c. somatostatin: regulates release of insulin and glucagon
33. a. Type 1 diabetes
    b. Type 2 diabetes

34. a. Glucose is unable to enter cells, causing hyperglycemia.
    b. Glucose accumulates in the bloodstream, causing an osmotic gradient to occur, which results in fluid moving from the intracellular to the extracellular space.
    c. Fluid is filtered through the glomerulus into the renal tubule; the renal tubule reabsorbs the glucose and most of the water in the filtrate; when glucose concentrate exceeds the threshold, the glucose is excreted in the urine.
    d. Water is also excreted as part of the osmotic diversion.
    e. Urinary fluid losses cause the individual to experience thirst.
    f. Because glucose is unable to enter the cells, the body burns fat for energy but also uses protein.
    g. The liver metabolizes protein and converts it to glucose for energy use, which contributes to hyperglycemia.
    h. Because the body cannot use glucose, and fat and protein stores are depleted, the patient experiences hunger and increased food intake, further elevating blood glucose.
    i. When fats are metabolized, they are broken down into fatty acids and ketone bodies; the ketone bodies are used as a source of fuel for glucose, and the excess is excreted in the urine and in the lungs.
    j. The production of ketone bodies (which are organic acids) and the dehydration that results from the osmotic diuresis lead to a metabolic acidosis.
35. a. microvascular changes
    (1) nephropathy
    (2) retinopathy
    (3) neuropathy
36. polyphagia, polydipsia, polyuria
37. serum glucose levels
38. a. 3
    b. 2
    c. 1
    d. 4
39. Insulin pumps
40. Self-blood glucose monitoring
41. Glycosylated hemoglobin; 7.5%
42. lowers
43. a physiologic reflex response to a decreased blood glucose level, which results in release of stress hormones (epinephrine, growth hormone, and corticosteroids) and a rebound hyperglycemia
44. insulin reaction
45. diabetic ketoacidosis
46. a. rapid
    b. gradual
    c. imbalances in food intake, insulin, and activity
    d. illness, growth, emotional upset, too much food, or inaccurate or missed insulin doses
    e. lability of mood; difficulty concentrating; shaky feeling; pallor; sweating; shallow respirations; tremors; tachycardia
    f. lethargic; dulled sensorium; increased thirst; signs of dehydration; acetone breath; rapid and deep respirations; weak pulse; diminished reflexes; nausea/vomiting; flushed skin
    g. shock; coma; death
    h. acidosis; coma; death
    i. glucose negative; acetone negative; output normal
    j. glucose positive; acetone positive; early polyuria, late oliguria
    k. decreased: 60 mg per 100 ml, or less
    l. increased: 250 mg per 100 ml, or more
47. sugar
48. to enhance absorption
49. adolescent

Applying Critical Thinking to Nursing Practice

A.
1. a. short stature but proportional height and weight
    b. growth measurement below 5th percentile
    c. height may be retarded more than weight
    d. appears well nourished
    e. skeletal proportions normal
    f. tends to be relatively inactive and shuns aggressive sports
    g. retarded bone-age in proportion to height-age
    h. eruption of permanent teeth delayed
    i. teeth overcrowded and malpositioned
    j. sexual development delayed but normal
    k. premature aging in later life
2. a. overgrowth of long bones; may reach a height of 8 feet
    b. rapid and increased development of muscles and viscera
    c. weight increased but in proportion to height
    d. proportional enlargement of head circumference
3. a. polyuria
    b. polydipsia
    c. irritability
    d. dehydration signs
4. cessation or retardation of growth in an infant whose growth has previously been normal
5. early identification of children with hypothyroidism
6. a. instituting seizure precautions
    b. instituting safety precautions
    c. reducing environmental stimuli
    d. observing for signs of laryngospasm
B.
1. to monitor for hyperpyrexia and shocklike state
2. Overdosage can precipitate complications.
3. weakness, poor muscle control, paralysis, cardiac dysrhythmias, and apnea
C.
1. immediate recognition of ambiguous genitalia in the newborn
2. to suppress the abnormally high secretion of adrenocorticotropic hormone
D.
1. a. (1) rapid assessment
        (2) adequate insulin to reduce the elevated blood
        (3) fluids to overcome dehydration
        (4) electrolyte replacement (especially potassium)
    b. Child exhibits adequate hydration.
2. blood glucose monitoring
3. ensure day-to-day consistency in total calorie, protein, fat, and carbohydrate
4. a. irritability, shaky feeling, sweating, pallor, tremors, tachycardia, shallow respirations
    b. Give the child simple sugar.
5. a. Child will learn to conduct blood glucose monitoring.
    b. Child and family will be able to interpret results of glucose monitoring.
    c. Child and family will learn the care and maintenance of monitoring equipment.
6. so that the child and family can learn how to adjust insulin, based on blood glucose level
7. Child takes responsibility for management of disease commensurate with age and capabilities.
E.
1. a. Child will accept teaching provided.
    b. Child will demonstrate understanding of disease and its therapy.
    c. Child will demonstrate understanding of meal planning.
    d. Child will demonstrate knowledge of and ability to administer insulin.

e. Child will demonstrate ability to test blood glucose level and urine.
f. Child will demonstrate understanding of proper hygiene.
g. Child will demonstrate understanding of importance of exercise regimen.
h. Child will demonstrate understanding and management of hyperglycemia and hypoglycemia.
i. Child will wear medical identification.
j. Child will keep proper records of insulin administration and testing procedures.
k. Child will engage in self-management.

Chapter 30

Review of Essential Concepts

1. true
2. a. contact with injurious agents such as infectious organisms, toxic chemicals, and physical trauma
   b. hereditary factors
   c. external factors that produce a reaction in the skin (e.g., allergens)
   d. a systemic disease in which the lesions are a cutaneous manifestation
3. a. 2
   b. 4
   c. 1
   d. 3
4. a. 4
   b. 2
   c. 1
   d. 5
   e. 3
   f. 8
   g. 7
   h. 6
   i. 9
5. structural or physiologic disruptions of the integument that call for normal or abnormal tissue repair responses
6. a. superficial
   b. partial-thickness
   c. full-thickness
7. a. hemostasis
   b. inflammation
   c. proliferation
   d. remodeling
8. a. to prevent further damage
   b. to eliminate the cause of the damage
   c. to prevent complications
   d. to provide relief from discomfort while tissues undergo healing
9. moist wound
10. aggravate
11. c
12. inspection, palpation
13. increased erythema, edema, purulent exudate, pain, increased temperature
14. color, drainage, odor, necrosis, granulation tissue, fibrin slough, condition of wound edges, and color of surrounding skin
15. pruritus
16. Cool the skin by evaporation, relieve itching and inflammation, and cleanse the area by loosening and removing crusts and debris.

17. oatmeal, mineral oil
18. false
19. a. to prevent the spread of infection
    b. to prevent complications
20. a. administering parenteral antibiotics
    b. applying compresses
21. a. with inflammation and vesiculation
    b. by proliferating to form growths
22. griseofulvin
23. an inflammatory reaction of the skin to chemical substances, natural or synthetic, that evoke a hypersensitivity response, or to those agents that cause direct irritation
24. prevent further exposure of the skin to the offending substance
25. false
26. d
27. Further doses of the medication should be withheld and the rash reported to the attending physician.
28. a. interdigital surfaces
    b. axillary-cubital area
    c. popliteal folds
    d. inguinal region
29. permethrin 5% cream (Elimite)
30. b
31. epinephrine
32. to educate parents to protect their children from exposure to ticks
33. true
34. urine, feces, soaps, detergents, ointments, and friction
35. a. minimize skin wetness
    b. allow the skin to maintain its normal acidic pH
    c. minimize the interaction of urine and feces on skin
36. a. 2
    b. 1
    c. 3
37. a. to hydrate the skin
    b. to relieve pruritis
    c. to reduce the inflammation
    d. to prevent or control secondary infection
38. tacrolimus, pimecrolimus
39. a chronic, recurrent, inflammatory reaction of the skin, manifesting in thick, yellowish, scaly lesions
40. acne vulgaris
41. b
42. tretinoin (retin-A), benzoyl peroxide
43. side effects
44. a. percentage of the body surface area burned
    b. depth of the injury
45. d
46. Anemia is caused by direct heat destruction of red blood cells, hemolysis of injured red cells, and trapping of red cells in the microvascular thrombi of damaged cells.
47. hypoxia
48. a. to establish and maintain an adequate airway
    b. to establish a lifeline for fluid replacement therapy
    c. to maintain balanced nutrition
    d. to manage pain
49. a. to compensate for water and sodium lost to traumatized areas and interstitial spaces
    b. to reestablish sodium balance
    c. to restore circulating volume

    d. to provide adequate perfusion

    e. to correct acidosis

    f. to improve renal function

50. the infection rate and threat of sepsis

51. a. A topical antimicrobial ointment is applied directly to the wound surface, but the wound is left uncovered.

    b. An antimicrobial ointment is applied to gauze or directly to the wound; multiple layers of bulky gauze are placed over the primary layer and secured with gauze or net.

52. tissues obtained from human cadavers that are free from disease

53. a. Child will experience reduction of pain.

    b. Child will exhibit evidence of wound healing.

    c. Child will receive adequate nutrition and will achieve reduction in metabolic losses.

    d. Child will not experience complications during acute care.

    e. Child will not experience complications during long-term care.

    f. Child and family will receive emotional support.

54. scar formation

55. Protection

56. sufficient exposure that heat loss to local tissues allows small ice crystals to form in tissues, resulting in variable degrees of tissue loss and function

Applying Critical Thinking to Nursing Practice

A.

1. a. Child will experience no or minimal pruritis.

    b. Child will receive appropriate treatment for skin hydration.

    c. Child will experience no complications.

    d. Child and family will receive adequate support.

2. a. impaired skin integrity related to eczematous lesions

    b. risk for infection related to risk for secondary infection of primary lesions

    c. interrupted family processes related to child's discomfort and lengthy therapy

B.

1. The nurse assessed Sean's skin and noted the presence of a rash on the convex surfaces of the diaper area.

2. the wetness, pH, and fecal irritants

3. a. Use superabsorbent disposable diapers.

    b. Change diapers as soon as they become wet or soiled.

    c. Expose the area to light and air.

    d. Do not use rubber pants.

    e. Clean the area well after each soiling.

    f. Use an occlusive ointment.

    g. Avoid over-washing skin.

C.

1. because of their social nature and proximity to other children

2. the crawling insect and the insect's saliva on the skin

3. Nix, Rid

4. a. parental education

    b. prevention of reinfestation

D.

1. a. Position for minimal mechanical disturbance of graft site.

    b. Place patient on low air-loss bed; turn every 2 hours.

    c. Restrain if necessary.

    d. Maintain splints or dressings.

    e. Observe grafts for evidence of hematoma/fluid accumulation; aspirate or express fluids.

2. Adequate fluid resuscitation is maintained as evidenced by adequate tissue perfusion and maintenance of urine output.

3. to minimize exposure to infectious agents
4. altered nutrition (less than body requirements) related to loss of appetite
5. to maintain optimum joint and muscle function
6. The family demonstrates an understanding of the needs of the child and the impact the child's condition will have on them. Family sets realistic goals for selves, child, and others.

Chapter 31

Review of Essential Concepts

1. muscle activity
2. the functioning of other systems that may be affected secondarily—for example, the circulatory, renal, respiratory, muscular, and gastrointestinal systems
3. a. damage to the soft tissue, subcutaneous structures, and muscle
   b. occurs when the force of stress on the ligament is so great that it displaces the normal position of the opposing bone ends or the bone end to its socket
   c. occurs when trauma to a joint is so severe that a ligament is partially or completely torn or stretched by the force created as a joint is twisted or wrenched, often accompanied by damage to associated blood vessels, muscles, tendons, and nerves
   d. microscopic tear to the musculotendinous unit; has features in common with sprains
4. a. rest
   b. ice
   c. compression
   d. elevation
5. a. bend: a child's flexible bone can be bent 45° or more before breaking
   b. buckle fracture: compression of the porous bone; appears as raised or bulging projection at the fracture site
   c. greenstick fracture: occurs when a bone is angulated beyond the limits of bending
   d. complete fracture: divides the bone fragments with or without a periosteal hinge
6. a. to regain alignment and length of the bony fragments (reduction)
   b. to retain alignment and length (immobilization)
   c. to restore function to the injured parts
   d. to prevent further injury
7. traction, closed manipulation
8. pain, swelling, discoloration of exposed portions, decreased pulses, decreased temperature, or inability to move the exposed parts
9. a. to fatigue the involved muscle and reduce muscle spasm so that bones can be realigned
   b. to position the distal and proximal bone ends in desired realignment to promote satisfactory bone healing
   c. to immobilize the fracture site until realignment has been achieved and sufficient healing has taken place to permit casting or splinting
10. a. manual traction
    b. skin traction
    c. skeletal traction
11. a. 3
    b. 4
    c. 2
    d. 1
12. A severed part should be rinsed with normal saline; the limb should be wrapped loosely in sterile gauze and placed in a watertight plastic bag; cool the bag without freezing in ice water (do not pack in ice); label the bag with the child's name, date, and time; and transport the child to the hospital.
13. a. acetabular dysplasia or preluxation
    b. subluxation
    c. dislocation

14. Ortolani, Barlow
15. a. 4
    b. 1
    c. 2
    d. 3
16. a. correction of the deformity
    b. maintenance of the correction until normal muscle balance regained
    c. follow-up observation to avert possible recurrence
17. heterogenous group-inherited syndrome
18. a. avascular
    b. fragmentation or revascularization
    c. reparative
    d. regenerative
19. a spinal deformity in three planes, involving lateral curvature, spinal rotation causing rib asymmetry, and thoracic hypokyphosis
20. bracing, surgical spinal fusion
21. Bracing, exercise
22. internal fixation, instrumentation
23. The advantage to this procedure is that the patient can be mobile within a few days, and no postoperative immobilization is required.
24. log-rolled
25. infectious process of bone, exogenous, hematogenous
26. intravenous therapy, antibiotic
27. bed rest, immobilized
28. osteogenic sarcoma, Ewing sarcoma
29. a. arises in the metaphysis of long bones, usually lower extremities
    b. arises in the marrow spaces of the bones (usually long bones)
    c. radical surgical amputation followed by intensive chemotherapy
    d. intensive radiation of the involved bone combined with chemotherapy
30. prosthesis
31. rhabdomyosarcoma
32. orbit
33. false
34. a. to control pain
    b. to preserve joint range of motion and function
    c. to minimize effects of inflammation, such as joint deformity
    d. to promote normal growth and development
35. a. nonsteroidal antiinflammatory drugs (NSAIDS)
    b. methotrexate
    c. corticosteroids
    d. tumor necrosis factor inhibitor
36. Corticosteroids are not the drug of choice because of their chronic and serious side effect on growth.
37. a chronic, multisystem, autoimmune disease of the connective tissues and blood vessels, characterized by inflammation in potentially any body tissue
38. a classic photosensitive erythematous butterfly rash extending across nose and cheeks
39. a. Balance the medications necessary to avoid exacerbation and complications.
    b. Prevent or minimize treatment-associated morbidity.
40. The principal drugs are corticosteroids.
41. to help the child and family positively adjust to the disease and therapy

Applying Critical Thinking to Nursing Practice

A.
 1. to prevent dependent edema and to stimulate circulation, respiratory function, gastrointestinal motility, and neurologic sensations
 2. a. allow child to plan daily routine
    b. allow child to select diet
    c. allow child to choose own street clothes
    d. allow child to be as active in their care as possible
B.
 1. a. Keep the extremity elevated on pillows for the first day.
    b. Avoid indenting the cast until it is thoroughly dry.
    c. Encourage frequent rest for a few days, keeping the injured extremity elevated while resting.
    d. Avoid allowing the affected limb to hang down for any length of time.
 2. a. Do not allow the child to put anything in the cast.
    b. Keep a clear path for ambulation.
    c. Use crutches appropriately.
C.
 1. a. Understand the purpose of traction.
    b. Check the desired line of pull frequently and the relationship of distal fragment to proximal fragment.
    c. Check the function of component parts.
    d. Make sure ropes move freely through pulleys.
    e. Make sure weights hang freely.
    f. Maintain total body alignment and bed position.
    g. Do not remove traction.
 2. a. Observe for correct body alignment.
    b. Check after child has moved.
    c. Apply restraints when indicated.
    d. Maintain correct angles at joints.
D.
 1. a. leg shortening on affected side
    b. asymmetry of the thigh and gluteal fold
    c. limited abduction of hip on affected side
    d. positive Ortolani test
    e. positive Barlow test
 2. early, age, dysplasia
 3. a. Teach parents to apply and maintain the reduction device.
    b. Assess skin under harness for irritation daily.
    c. Avoid use of powders and lotions.
    d. Caution against unsupervised adjustment of harness.
    e. Help devise means for maintaining cleanliness.
E.
 1. a. body image disturbance related to the defect in body structure
    b. self-esteem disturbance related to immobility
 2. a. Accentuate positive aspects of appearance.
    b. Encourage Jane to wear attractive clothes and hairstyle.
    c. Emphasize positive long-term outcome.
    d. Help devise positive ways to deal with reactions of others.
 3. opioids administered through patient-controlled analgesia (PCA)
F.
 1. He would appear very ill; would be irritable and restless; and would have an elevated temperature, rapid pulse, and signs of dehydration. He would complain of localized tenderness, increased warmth, and diffuse swelling over the involved bone. The extremity would be painful, especially upon movement, and the child would hold it in semiflexion. The surrounding muscles are tense and resist passive movement.

2. a. Monitor intravenous equipment.
   b. Monitor intravenous site.
   c. Determine compatibility of antibiotics before administration.
   d. Take measures to protect the intravenous tubing from dislodgment.
G.
  1. nonsteroidal antiinflammatory drugs; fewer side effects, easier to administer, and very effective
  2. a. chronic pain related to joint inflammantion
     b. impaired physical mobility related to joint discomfort and stiffness
     c. bathing/hygiene, dressing/grooming, feeding, or toileting self-care deficit related to impaired joint mobility
     d. altered family processes related to a situational crisis (child with a chronic illness)
  3. Child is able to move with minimum or no discomfort.

Chapter 32

Review of Essential Concepts

1. a nonspecific term applied to disorders characterized by early-onset impaired movement and posture. It is nonprogressive and may be accompanied by perceptual problems, language deficits, and intellectual impairment.
2. No
3. a. spastic cerebral palsy: hypertonicity with poor control of posture, balance, and coordinated motion
   b. dyskinetic cerebral palsy: abnormal involuntary movements, athetosis
   c. ataxic cerebral palsy: wide-based gait; rapid, repetitive movements performed poorly
   d. mixed-type cerebral palsy: a combination of spasticity and athetosis
4. a. poor head control after 3 months of age
   b. stiff or rigid arms or legs
   c. pushing away or arching back
   d. floppy or limp body posture
   e. cannot sit up without support by 8 months of age
   f. uses only one side of the body or only the arms to crawl
5. Mental retardation may or may not be present.
6. a. to establish locomotion, communication, and self-help
   b. to gain optimum appearance and integration of motor functions
   c. to correct associated defects as effectively as possible
   d. to provide educational opportunities adapted to the needs and capabilities of the individual child
   e. to promote socialization experiences with other affected and unaffected children
7. Botox, baclofen (Lioresal)
8. d
9. b
10. a. prevention of latex allergy
    b. identification of children with a known hypersensitivity
11. a disorder characterized by progressive weakness and wasting of skeletal muscles
12. muscle fibers; progressive weakness and wasting of symmetric groups of skeletal muscles, with increasing disability and deformity
13. muscle groups affected, age of onset, rate of progression, and inheritance patterns
14. pseudohypertrophic muscular dystrophy or Duchenne muscular dystrophy (DMD)
15. respiratory or cardiac failure
16. a. Maintain optimal function of all muscles.
    b. Prevent contractures.
17. acute demyelinating polyneuropathy with a progressive, usually ascending, flaccid paralysis
18. assisted ventilation

19. an acute, preventable, and often fatal disease caused by an exotoxin produced by *Clostridium tetani*, an anaerobic, spore-forming, gram-positive bacillus
20. immune status, injury
21. tetanus immune globulin (TIG) and tetanus toxoid
22. ingestion of spores or vegetative cells of *Clostridium botulinum* and the subsequent release of the toxin from organisms colonizing in the gastrointestinal tract
23. honey, light or dark corn syrup
24. clinical history, physical examination, and laboratory detection of toxin or the organism in the patient's blood or stool
25. a. complete or partial paralysis of the lower extremities
    b. no functional use of any of the four extremities
26. a. maintenance of airway patency
    b. prevention of complications
    c. maintenance of function
27. functional electrical stimulation (FES)

Applying Critical Thinking to Nursing Practice

A.
1. a. Child will acquire mobility within personal capabilities.
   b. Child will acquire communication skills or use appropriate assistive devices.
   c. Child will engage in self-help activities.
   d. Child will receive appropriate education.
   e. Child will develop a positive self-image.
   f. Family will receive appropriate education and support in its efforts to meet the child's needs.
   g. Child will receive appropriate care if hospitalized.
2. a. Child will engage in self-help activities of daily living.
   b. Child engages in self-help activities commensurate with capabilities.
3. because children are sensitive to affective attitude of the professional
4. a. Child will receive optimum rest.
   b. Child will maintain good general health.

B.
1. a. Infant will not experience damage to the myelomeningocele sac.
   b. Infant will not experience complications.
   c. Family will receive support and education.
2. a. The myelomeningocele sac sustains no damage.
   b. The child exhibits no evidence of complications.
   c. The family members discuss their feelings and concerns and participate in the infant's care.
3. a. Reduce exposure to latex from birth on.
   b. Provide a latex-free environment to avoid all contact.

C.
1. Help parents develop a balance between limiting the child's activity because of muscular weakness and allowing the child to accomplish things by himself or herself.
2. encouraging parents to seek genetic counseling

D.
1. to prevent complications of the disease
2. Any two of the following are acceptable:
   Observe for difficulty in swallowing and for respiratory involvement
   Take frequent vital signs
   Monitor level of consciousness
   Maintain good postural alignment
   Change position frequently
   Perform passive range of motion every 4 hours
   Ensure adequate nutrition
   Provide bowel and bladder care to prevent constipation and urine retention

E.
1. baseline for neurologic functioning
2. preparing the child and family to live at home and function as independently as possible